Feed Me I'm Yours

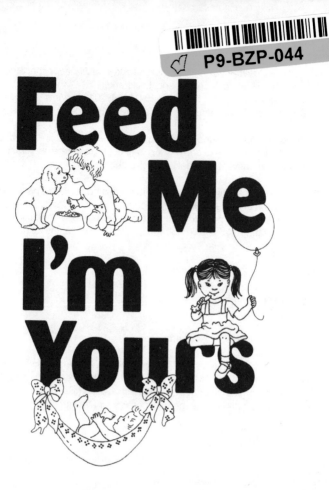

Vicki Lansky

Illustrated by Kathy Rogers

Da Capo
LIFE
LONG

Da Capo Press
Hachette Book Group
1290 Avenue of the Americas, New York, NY 10104
www.dacapopress.com
@DaCapoPress

Printed in the United States of America

This book was first written in 1974 by six mothers, all members of the Childbirth
Education Association of Minneapolis–St. Paul, which is now the headquarters
of the International Childbirth Education Association (ICEA). ICEA is a nonprofit
organization that prepares expectant parents for a rewarding childbirth
experience.

First Edition: October 1974

Current Revised Edition: August 2013

Published by Da Capo Lifelong Books, an imprint of Perseus Books, LLC, a
subsidiary of Hachette Book Group, Inc. The Da Capo Lifelong name and logo
are trademarks of the Hachette Book Group.

The publisher is not responsible for websites (or their content) that are not
owned by the publisher.

Cover design by Nancy Tuminelly and Tamara Peterson

Library of Congress cataloging information is on file.

ISBNs: 978-0-684-02862-0 (paperback), 978-1-451-61598-2 (e-book)

LSC-C

10 9 8 7 6 5 4 3 2

Dedication

To parents everywhere, from those of us who've been there and wish we knew then what we know now.

In the beginning, you'll be choosing between breastfeeding and formula. The field of food choices widens significantly by the time your child is six months old, and for the next few years the responsibility for your child's food selection is mainly yours.

With this recipe book, we've tried to help you with that selection. Our recipes and ideas have been collected for their nutrition, convenience, and fun. We hope this book will ease your task of meal preparation and help you enjoy your infant, toddler, or preschooler.

Vicki Lansky
and Jill Jacobson
Stephanie Keane
Norine Larson
Mary Popehn
Lois Parker

Thirty Years Later...

In 1974 I was a young mother at home in suburban Minneapolis with two small children, ages one and three. I had majored in art history in college and worked as a sportswear buyer in New York City before getting married and starting a family. I had no experience with writing and publishing. But then I had an idea for a small cookbook that could be a fundraiser for a local childbirth education group. With input from five other mothers in a total of two group meetings (with at least half a dozen children in tow at each meeting), I created a cookbook for new mothers. The only title ever suggested—*Feed Me! I'm Yours*—was casually thrown out at one of those meetings. As they say, the rest is history.

The first hand-typed, hand-collated edition of *Feed Me! I'm Yours*, with a black-and-white photo of my baby girl on its cover, was published in November 1974. The food editor of the Minneapolis paper gave us a wonderful review in the Sunday edition that Thanksgiving weekend, and we were flooded with orders. A few weeks later I remarked that many people were reordering additional copies. Suddenly my husband's ears perked up. He realized that reorders were a different breed of sales from initial orders. My evening project took on new interest to him. Within a few months we formed Meadowbrook Press (because we lived on Meadowbrook Lane), learned about typesetting and printing estimates, and became the publishers of *Feed Me! I'm Yours*.

Over the next year we learned how to publicize and market this new "infant" we had produced. My husband convinced local media to interview me and local bookstores to buy the book. I went on TV talk shows to demonstrate how easy it was to make baby food from scratch, taking time from madly invoicing and delivering copies of the book to those bookstores. We learned how to sell copies beyond Minneapolis. One successful strategy was our "relative marketing plan." We went to bookstores in markets where our relatives lived so we could afford to stay while we publicized the book.

Whatever we did seemed to work. We seemed to be in the right place at the right time. Commercial baby food was under attack, and I represented mothers who wanted alternatives that were easy and practical. We were forced to prove ourselves market by market, which we did. Today, family topic TV is dominated by a handful of syndicated shows. This was not the case in the late seventies. Major cities had local talk shows that wanted the type of information I offered. To reach them, I was forced to travel.

After we had sold over a hundred thousand copies of *Feed Me!* from our house, Bantam Books offered to publish a mass-market paperback edition while we continued to publish the spiral-bound edition. With Bantam's credibility behind us, we were able to set up my appearance on *The Phil Donahue Show* (then broadcast out of Chicago), which boosted sales tremendously. Counting both editions, more than three million copies have been sold to date.

I'm proud that *Feed Me! I'm Yours* remains a valuable resource for parents. I have updated this new edition to make sure you benefit from current information, but it's still basically the same book that has served so many parents over the years. It had become a classic baby food cookbook and one of the Horatio Alger stories in the publishing community. It was my first book, and I thought my last. I was wrong. Another twenty-four parenting books followed, plus five household hints books. (I graduated from writing parenting tips to writing household tips in 1988, thanks to *Family Circle* magazine.) No one has been more amazed than I.

My two children, now in their thirties, have had the good grace to turn out well—for which I am grateful—*for there are no guarantees in this unique business of raising children.* Not only have they helped my credibility, they have been a remarkable gift. They are my credentials, my graduate degree, as well as my pride and joy. They have even developed good eating habits, which I will not presume to take all the credit for—only some of it.

Now I'm a grandmother, and it's a joy to watch my children take pride in passing on good eating habits to the next generation.

Vicki Lansky
Fall 2004
www.practicalparenting.com

Contents

Introduction

Welcome to the world of the "haves" (people who have children, that is) and those umpteen new responsibilities, joys, anxieties, precious moments, and sleepless nights.

With your first child comes a new and demanding role: nurturing a totally dependent person. What you feed your child helps determine his or her mental and physical health. No one food contains all the nutrients we need, in the amounts we need, so we must opt for a variety of foods representing the different food groups, including:

- Grains (including breads, cereals, pasta, and rice)
- Vegetables
- Fruits
- Dairy (including milk, cheese, and yogurt)
- Protein foods (including fish, poultry, eggs, dry beans, and nuts)

Fats and sweets are not actually a food group. (They come "with" servings from other food groups.)

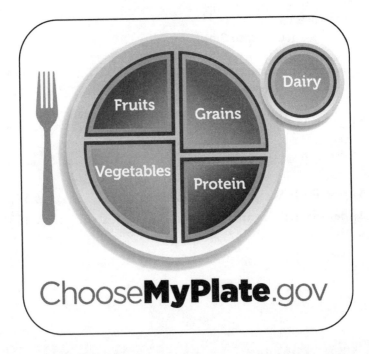

ChooseMyPlate.gov

Below are sample servings for a four-to-six-year-old. Two- to three-year-olds should be offered smaller serving sizes.

- *Grain group:* 1 slice of bread; ½ cup of cooked rice or pasta; ½ cup of cooked cereal; 1 ounce of ready-to-eat cereal
- *Vegetable group:* ½ cup of chopped raw (or cooked) vegetables; 1 cup of raw leafy vegetables
- *Fruit group:* 1 piece of fruit or melon wedge; ¾ cup of juice; ½ cup of canned fruit; ¼ cup of dried fruit
- *Dairy group:* 1 cup of milk or yogurt; 2 ounces of cheese
- *Protein group:* 2–3 ounces of cooked lean meat, poultry, or fish; (½ cup cooked dry beans or 1 egg counts as 1 ounce of lean meat; 2 tablespoons of peanut butter count as 1 ounce of meat.)

We are aware of the need to limit large amounts of fats and sweets in a child's diet, but remember that fats are necessary for early growth and development.

A good diet is low in refined carbohydrates and sugars. Natural carbohydrates and sugars appear in fruits, flours, cereal, and vegetables. If your child's diet is varied and the quantity intakes are appropriate, your child's body will get what it needs.

Americans are often overfed but undernourished. The American diet contains far more calories than the body needs. The empty calories in foods made primarily of refined sugars squeeze the nutritious foods out of a more healthful diet. And even when we think we're watching our sugar intake, many of the grocery products we buy contain hidden sugars. Beware of what goes into those nice, consumer-oriented packages; read the labels of foods you buy.

Nurturing includes providing a balanced and varied diet for your child, not determining the quantities that should be eaten. Children's appetites change with their growth patterns. Each child's metabolism is different, with its own food requirements. Children come in many sizes and shapes. There are times when they have more body fat than at other times. This is normal. Your child will eat as much as his or her system demands at any time if you provide enough varied food at appropriate intervals. Only when your children are old enough to buy junk food must you take care that nutritious foods aren't pushed out of their diets.

Your attitude toward food can encourage your child to develop a healthy attitude and lifelong good habits. In fact, your attitude is the key to feeding this new child of yours.

> Be flexible. Respect strong food dislikes. And remember, love is not equal to the amount of food your child eats.

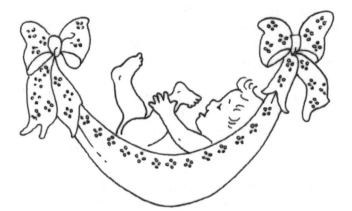

Chapter One
Baby Food

Economy, increased nutritional awareness, and concerns about processed foods are some of the reasons why many parents are making their own baby food. Others are discovering that making baby food at home is much simpler and less time consuming than they'd imagined. It can be gratifying to provide your infant with meals that save money (up to 50 percent), are free of additives and fillers, and are as fresh and nutritious as the foods you serve the rest of your family.

Homemade versus Store-Bought

You don't have to be a purist to make your own baby food. You might be using some commercial baby foods, so when you purchase those little jars, read the labels carefully. Stay with the basic fruits, vegetables, and strained meats. Avoid blends and dinners since you get fewer nutrients per serving than if you combine single-ingredient jars. Avoid jars containing added sugar, salt, and modified starches. Forget the baby desserts; babies don't need them any more than we do.

Baby food in jars is preserved through the canning method. No preservatives are added. What is added is to help the color and texture appeal for the adult buying it and feeding it to a baby.

Stores have responded to parents' interest in organic baby food. In jars you can find brands such as Earth's Best, Healthy Times, and Organic Baby. Even Gerber has an organic line of baby foods called Tender Harvest. Heinz has also added a brand called Nature's Goodness. (See Appendix II for more information.) Most of these are still made with added water and fillers, such as flour, though the water may be filtered and the flour may be organic. Just because it's organic doesn't mean you don't have to read the label. Organic baby foods cost more, but if your baby likes them better, then they're probably worth it.

You can store previously opened jars of commercial baby food in the refrigerator for two or three days. Commercial baby food manufacturers do not recommend using the container as a serving dish because the baby's saliva on the spoon contaminates the food in the jar and speeds up the spoiling process. Another reason to avoid feeding a baby directly from the jar is the tendency to finish the jar and thus overfeed your baby. Plus, by transferring baby food from its jar to a serving dish, you can check the product for any foreign matter.

Homemade Baby Food

The most commonly recommended first food is baby instant rice cereal. It's rarely allergenic and should be iron-fortified. If you're nervous about making your own baby food, start with some of the many soft or puréed grocery-store foods available to you down the *other* aisles. These include unsweetened applesauce, canned pumpkin, banana (the riper it is, the more digestible it is), Cream of Rice cereal, and after about ten months, plain yogurt and cottage cheese (which may need a little extra mashing). A mashed baked potato thinned with breast milk or formula is also a fine first food.

When to Start

Don't be in a hurry to start your baby on solid foods. Milk (either breast milk or formula) provides all the nutrients your baby needs for the first four to six months and continues to be very important throughout the first year. Current guidelines suggest breastfeeding for at least one year. While "breast is best," the American Academy of Pediatrics recommends that babies on formula drink an iron-fortified brand until they're twelve months old. When solid foods are initially introduced at four to six months, they supplement—but don't replace—breast milk or formula.

Microwaving Bottles: Safety Tips

DON'T microwave breast milk. Instead, thaw or warm it up by running lukewarm water over the bottle or setting the bottle in a pan of warm water. Heating breast milk in a microwave is believed to reduce its anti-infective properties.

DON'T microwave formula in a glass bottle (as the glass could crack) or in colored plastic bottles (unless they're labeled microwave safe).

DO use clear plastic bottles—without bottle liners—when heating formula. As a general guideline, heat a cold eight ounces on high for about 45 seconds. Leave the bottle uncovered in the microwave to allow heat to escape.

REMEMBER that microwaves can heat liquids unevenly, so invert (don't shake) a warmed bottle (with nipple replaced) about ten times to distribute the heat. Then test a few drops of the heated liquid on the back of your hand to check its temperature.

Some parents introduce a bit of cereal at bedtime, on the recommendation of a friend or relative, to help a baby sleep through the night. There's no conclusive evidence from academic circles that this works—but there's no evidence that it doesn't work, either. We do know that an infant will not benefit nutritionally from cereal and that a baby's digestive tract is usually not ready for cereals or *any solids* until four to six months of age. Introducing solids earlier than four to six months is believed to increase a child's risk of developing type 1 diabetes, allergies, and weight issues later in life.

The introduction of solid foods is a red-letter day. Your child may not be grateful or even cooperative at first, but don't worry. If you find yourself spooning food into a mouth that's pushing it back out, then your baby is still in the tongue-thrust reflex stage and isn't ready for solid foods. Read this as a message from your baby's body, not as a rejection of your fine efforts. Wait a week and try again. Don't be in a hurry. (Think of the time and money you'll save!)

On the other hand, if your baby is grabbing food off your plate, it's time to start new foods and textures. (Actually, you're probably a bit late.)

How to Start

Check with your baby's doctor before introducing new foods. Introduce them to your baby one at a time, at four-to-five-day intervals, so you can determine if they're the source of any allergic reaction. Offer new foods late in the morning or at midday, so you can monitor your baby's response during the afternoon and possibly avoid a sleepless night. A few spoonfuls at first will usually suffice. The idea is to introduce your baby to new tastes and textures—not to fill your baby up. Signs of food intolerance include vomiting, gassiness, diarrhea, watery eyes, skin rash, or hives. Remember, three meals a day is an adult pattern for our culture, not a necessary approach for babies.

Here are two good bits of advice:

- **Follow your doctor's preference.** Babies prosper under as many different schedules as there are doctors. You also have to live with your doctor. (If you have definite opinions on the subject, interview several doctors before choosing one.)
- **Follow your own instincts.** Babies prosper under as many different schedules as there are parents. (If, on the other hand, your baby is not prospering, return to the previous paragraph.)

Whether you give your baby solids before or after breast milk or formula depends on your baby's preference. Some babies need a little milk first to take the edge off their hunger so they can relax enough to be spoon-fed. Start by feeding solid foods once or twice a day in the morning or evening. Choose a time when your baby seems hungry or when you both need a change of pace.

Allergy Alert

Many doctors recommend withholding nuts (also a choking hazard), nut butters, egg white, citrus fruits, cow's milk, berries, soy, tomatoes, corn, fish, and even some wheat products until a child is past one year of age, as they may cause allergic reactions, especially in food-sensitive families.

Tools of the Trade

Something to Cook In

Clean pots and appliances (stove-top or oven) are all you need for cooking your baby's foods. A slow cooker, pressure cooker, and microwave can also be helpful. No, don't go out and buy them. Just use them if you have them.

Steaming fruits and vegetables is best because many nutrients are often lost in cooking water. Inexpensive steamer baskets that collapse to fit most pans work well, but make sure the pot you use has a tight-fitting lid to keep the steam in.

Cooking fruits and vegetables in a microwave is a form of steaming from the inside out and is an excellent way to cook small quantities quickly while preserving nutrients. Use only microwave-safe containers and covers. Stir foods well and test before serving, as foods can heat unevenly and create hot spots.

Something to Purée With

By puréeing the unseasoned food *you* eat, you'll accustom your baby to the table foods he or she will eat soon. A fork can be used to mash food, but some of the following might be more efficient:

- A **blender** can quickly and easily purée almost any food into the finest consistency. You'll find that vegetables purée best in larger quantities, and meats in smaller quantities. In general, you'll be using the highest speeds to create a fine purée for your younger baby. As your baby grows, you can proceed to slower speeds for a coarser consistency. Blenders are reasonably priced and useful for making other child-oriented foods, such as shakes and homemade peanut butter (for an older child). You can also use a blender to reconstitute powdered milk or frozen orange juice concentrate quickly, or to purée vegetables that can be hidden in meat loaf or spaghetti sauce.

- A **food processor** can also be used to purée foods for your baby. It's difficult to purée small amounts in a full-size food processor, so be prepared to do large quantities and freeze most of it. (For information on freezing baby food, see page 12.) Small food processors are also available now.

- A **standard food mill** can be purchased in a large or small size. You place food in the basket, and as you turn the handle, the blade presses food through holes in the bottom of the basket. The food mill strains most cooked foods to a smooth consistency. Meat, however, will have a slightly coarser texture.

- A **baby food grinder** (a smaller version of the food mill, but with reverse action) simplifies puréeing small amounts of fresh food for your baby. You put the food in the well and place the turning disc on top. As you turn the handle and press down, the puréed food comes to the top and can be served right from the grinder. The grinder's small size makes it convenient to take along when you travel or eat out. It will grind fruits, vegetables, and soft-cooked meats. The grinder also conveniently sifts out the hulls of peas and corn.

  After your baby outgrows the need for puréed food, you'll find the grinder convenient for chopping nuts, grinding raisins and other dried fruits, softening butter or margarine, making egg salad, mashing a banana, mashing a baked or boiled potato, grating soft cheese, and probably many more uses.

  Baby food grinders are usually found in the baby departments of retail baby stores and some discount stores—but *not* in kitchen stores. What used to be known as the Happy Baby Food Grinder is now called the Kidco Baby Food Mill. It costs under $20. (To find a retail store in your area, visit www.kidcoinc.com/dealers.cfm.) It's also available by catalog or online from One Step Ahead. (Call 800-274-8440 or visit www.onestepahead.com.)

Handling and Storing Foods

Proper handling is important when you make your own baby food because babies are more vulnerable to food-borne illnesses.

- Work with clean hands and clean utensils, *including clean grinders and cutting boards.*
- Scrub, peel, and seed fresh fruits and vegetables before cooking.

- Prepare a food immediately after removing it from the refrigerator, and freeze any leftovers or volume foods immediately.
- Serve, refrigerate, or freeze baby food immediately after preparing it.

Freezing Options

When you make more food than your baby will eat at one meal, you need a way to store it safely. Freezing your own baby food gives you the variety and convenience of commercially prepared baby food. You'll find it easy to cook in volume, and freezing large batches means you can always keep an adequate supply on hand. You'll never need to rush to prepare food for a hungry baby. You can easily freeze meal-size portions for your baby using one of two methods: food cubes or plops. As your baby's appetite grows, you can add more cubes per meal or make bigger plops.

The Food Cube Method: Pour cooked, puréed food into molded plastic (pop-out) ice cube trays. Freeze immediately. Pop out the frozen cubes and transfer them to plastic freezer bags. Label and date. The food cubes can be stored for up to two months.

The Plop Method: Plop cooked, puréed, or finely ground foods by the spoonful onto a baking sheet. The size of each plop depends on how much you think your baby will eat at one meal. Freeze immediately. Transfer frozen plops to plastic bags. Label and date. Plops can be stored for up to two months.

Before a meal, take out the food you want to serve. Thaw it in the refrigerator or warm it in a microwave or an egg-poacher cup over boiling water. Remember that cold food and milk are acceptable to your baby, even if not to you. Your baby's mouth is very sensitive, so foods that seem warm to you may seem hot to your baby.

A cube or plop travels well for short journeys. By the time you've arrived, your baby's meal is defrosted and ready to eat. Food can also be frozen in empty, clean baby food jars. Be careful not to fill them completely, because food will expand while freezing. Small, stackable plastic jars with lids can serve the same purpose. Or use snack-size plastic storage bags to freeze meal-size portions. Store protein foods, cereals, vegetables, and fruits in separate containers when freezing. Don't refreeze thawed foods.

Baby's Cereals

Cereals are typically the first foods given to babies because they're fortified with iron. You'll find the commercial instant baby cereals both convenient and nutritious. Instant rice cereal is commonly recommended since it's rarely allergenic. You can also prepare cereals such as Cream of Wheat, oatmeal, and Wheatena by running them through your blender before cooking. It pays to make these cereals in quantity and freeze the balance. (See page 12.)

Hints: When preparing cereals for your baby, keep in mind that:
- A nursing mother may add expressed breast milk to cereals (or any foods) to make them more readily accepted, as the smell and taste are familiar to the baby.
- Any cereal can be sweetened with puréed fruits that have been introduced safely.
- A little plain yogurt (with active cultures) can be added to hot cereal. It gives a creamy texture to grainy cereals.

Honey Alert

Avoid using honey and corn syrup in beverages and foods for infants younger than one year. There's concern that they may contain botulism spores that infants can't handle.

Baby's Fruits

All fresh fruits (except bananas, papayas, and avocados) must be cooked until they're soft before puréeing. Canned fruits packed in their own juice are cooked in the canning process and are easy to purée and serve. If they come in sugary syrup, drain and rinse the fruit before puréeing.

Bananas

Use one medium-size, fully ripe (speckled-skin) banana. The riper the banana, the more digestible it will be for your baby. Cut it in half and peel one half to use. Cover the remaining half in the peel and store it in the refrigerator for up to two days. Mash the half banana with a fork or put it through a baby food grinder. You can also peel ripe bananas, wrap them tightly in meal-size portions, and freeze. When ready to use, thaw and use immediately. (For an older baby who's ready for chunkier foods, you can feed a banana right out of the peel with a spoon, one small bite at a time.)

Cooking Fruits

Apples, peaches, pears, plums, apricots, and most other fruits can be prepared using one of the following methods:

Boiling: Wash fruit, peel, and cut into small pieces. Add 1 cup fruit to ¼ cup boiling water. Simmer until tender (10–20 minutes). Don't add sugar; babies prefer the natural sweetness of the fruit. Blend or purée until smooth. Refrigerate what you'll use that day and freeze the balance.

Steaming: Wash fruit, peel, and steam for 15–20 minutes. Cool. Remove core, seeds, or pits. Blend or purée until smooth. Refrigerate what you'll use that day and freeze the balance.

Microwaving: Wash one piece of fruit. Remove core or pit. Place in a small glass with 2–3 teaspoons of water. Cover lightly. Microwave 1–2 minutes until fruit is tender. Cool and peel. Mash or purée until smooth.

The following fruit combinations are good for older babies who enjoy textures.

Tropical Treat

½ very ripe avocado, mashed or puréed
½ very ripe banana, mashed or puréed
¼ cup cottage cheese or yogurt

Combine ingredients.

Cottage–Cheese Fruit

½ cup large-curd cottage cheese
½ cup fresh fruit, raw or cooked
4–6 tablespoons orange juice

Blend quickly and serve cool. You can use this recipe to incorporate one of your prepared fruits into a whole meal.

Monkey Mash

½ mashed banana
½ small mashed baked potato or yam

Mix well. If needed, add breast milk, formula, or a little water.

Homemade Fruit Gelatin

1 envelope unflavored gelatin
¼ cup warm water
1 cup puréed fruit

Dissolve gelatin in water. Stir in fruit and chill.

Baby's Vegetables

Fresh vegetables should be used whenever possible for best nutrition, flavor, and economy. Frozen vegetables are your best substitute for fresh. Canned vegetables, while not as nutritious, are still convenient and worthwhile, though they often have too much added salt. They're already cooked and need only be puréed. (Use the liquid from the can, if possible, because many nutrients are contained in it.)

Basic Vegetable Recipe

Cook beets, carrots, sweet potatoes, peas, green beans, potatoes, and most other vegetables using one of the following methods:

Boiling: Peel and slice fresh vegetables for fast cooking, or use frozen ones. Cook in ½–1 inch of water for 20 minutes or until tender. Purée or blend with some of the cooking water.

Steaming: Peel and slice fresh vegetables, or use frozen. Steam over boiling water until tender. Purée or blend with some cooking water to get the right consistency.

Microwaving: Peel, clean, and slice fresh vegetables, or use frozen. In a microwave-safe dish (with a touch of water), cook vegetables until tender. Potatoes need to be pierced several times first to allow interior steam to escape. Single potatoes generally cook in 3–5 minutes. Purée or blend with cooking water or add water if necessary.

Baked Sweet Potato and Apples

¾ cup cooked sweet potato
1 cup applesauce or apples (peeled, cored, and sliced)
¼ cup liquid (breast milk, formula, or water)

Preheat oven to 350°F. Mix sweet potatoes and apples in buttered baking dish. Pour liquid over mixture. Cover and bake for 30 minutes. Purée or mash with a fork.

Vegetable Soup

¼ cup cooked, puréed vegetables
1 teaspoon butter, margarine, or vegetable oil
1 tablespoon whole-wheat or white flour, or instant baby cereal
¼ cup liquid (water or broth)

Combine vegetables and oil in a saucepan and place on low heat. Mix cereal and liquid separately and gradually stir into vegetables. Heat until warm.

Baby's Meats

You can purée any unseasoned meat you've cooked for your family, or cook up to a month's supply of meat for your baby and purée it. If you want a smoother consistency, mix meat with a small serving of instant baby rice cereal and some breast milk or formula. Even a little water or juice will help puréeing. Combine chicken with a little banana and breast milk or formula to get a smooth texture. Meats cooked in a slow cooker (minus seasonings) are tender and easy to purée.

All-Purpose Meat Stew

1½ pounds stew meat (in 1-inch cubes)
⅓ cup flour
2 tablespoons vegetable oil
3 cups water
4 medium potatoes
5 medium carrots
1 10-ounce package frozen peas

Coat meat with flour and brown in oil. Add water and cover pan tightly. Simmer 1½ hours. Scrub, peel, and cube potatoes and carrots. Add to meat. Simmer 15 minutes. Add peas and simmer 5 minutes. Take out a serving for adults and purée the balance. Makes 4–5 cups.

Variation: Substitute any vegetable or ½ cup rice for potatoes.

Pineapple Chicken

canned pineapple packed in its own juice
boiled or baked chicken

Drain pineapple and combine with chicken in a blender. Purée to a consistency appropriate for your child. Freeze excess. For a snack drink, strain the drained juice, mix with water, and serve.

Cockadoodle Stew

1 cup cooked cubed chicken or turkey
¼ cup cooked rice
¼ cup cooked vegetables
¼ cup chicken broth
¼ cup breast milk or formula

Purée together and make food cubes or plops. (See page 12.)

As your child matures, remember that:
• Good substitutes for meat include large-curd cottage cheese, boneless fish, cheese, tofu, cooked egg yolks, macaroni and cheese, soft-cooked beans, and nut butters.
• Even puréed macaroni and cheese can be frozen for future needs.
• Foods like rice pudding, chicken noodle soup, and even chunky applesauce can help ease an older baby into foods with more substance and texture.

Skip the Salt

These recipes do not require extra salt. Studies indicate that excess salt contributes to hypertension later in life. Since a taste for salty food is acquired, you can help your child avoid this health risk by minimizing added salt in his or her diet.

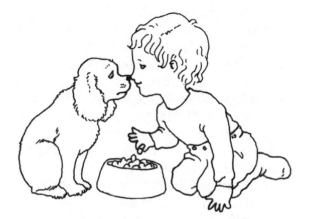

Chapter Two
Finger Foods

Good health depends on sound eating habits. What—and how—your child eats is established in the early years.

Introduce finger foods when your baby has enough eye-hand coordination to pick up objects with fingers or a spoon and get them into his or her mouth. At approximately six to eight months, when your baby is able to sit in a highchair and can reach for objects, a piece of graham cracker or a few Cheerios will be of great interest. If you allow your baby to experiment with foods (ignoring the mess), you'll have fewer problems in the long run. The more you allow your baby to do, the faster your baby will learn. Don't be surprised if you need two spoons for every meal—one for your baby and one for you!

Be sure you have the proper equipment: a highchair, a baby-size spoon (small enough to fit in your baby's mouth with a handle short enough for your baby to control), and a sippy cup with two handles (to save you time cleaning up the floor). Speaking of floors, you may want to use newspapers or a plastic tablecloth under the highchair.

Young children need far less food than many parents expect. A child eats when hungry and will take only what's needed to maintain a proper growth rate. Servings should be small, and so should plates or bowls. It's better to serve small portions first and second portions if needed than to be unhappy if a child hasn't finished a single large serving. Add new foods gradually. If your child rejects a particular food, return to a favorite and offer the new food again in a few days. It isn't always easy to respect your child's strong food dislikes, but it's important to try. Don't fret! Don't nag!

Sometime after one year of age, your child's appetite will decrease because the first-year growth spurt will slow down. Despite knowing this, it still comes as a surprise when children refuse to eat or finish foods they enjoyed or wolfed down just a week or month before. Toddlers change their food preferences from day to day and meal to meal, so remember to offer old favorites and previously refused foods from time to time. Some children cling to the personal service of being fed, but (given the opportunity) all children learn to feed themselves.

Common Choking Hazards for Babies and Toddlers

Hot dogs, whole or cut into circle slices
Grapes, whole
Carrots, raw
Hard candy
Meat chunks
Popcorn
Beans, raw

Cherries with pits
Nuts (also a common allergen)
Raisins
Olives, whole
Fish bones
Ice cubes

Use caution when serving toast sticks, bread sticks, and raw carrot sticks to young toddlers. Appropriateness will vary depending on whether a child has molars. Also, peanut butter should be used sparingly (if at all) or thinned with milk for young toddlers so it won't stick to the back of the mouth and cause choking.

Some children are more susceptible to choking than others, but all children have smaller air passages and weaker gag reflexes than adults. Finger foods should be eaten only when your child is sitting up—not while running and not while lying down—and only with adult supervision.

Finger Foods for Babies Six to Nine Months Old

Avocado, ripe
Arrowroot cookies
Bananas, mashed or in small pieces
Canned pears and peaches
Cereals, cooked
Cheerios or other unsweetened dry cereals
Chicken liver and other tender meat, mashed or chopped
Graham crackers
Ground meat
Potatoes, mashed
Pudding
Soda crackers
Soft-cooked vegetables, mashed

Finger Foods for Babies Ten Months to One Year Old

Bagels, soft
Carrots and other vegetables, cooked soft
Cheeses, soft
Chicken, in soft-cooked pieces
Cottage cheese, preferably large-curd
Eggs, boiled, scrambled (with breast milk, formula, or water), or poached (yolks only)
Egg noodles
Fish, without bones, including gefilte fish
Fresh toast "fingers," sliced in strips
Fruit cocktail, canned in its own juice
Kiwi, peeled

Macaroni and pastas, in interesting colors and shapes
Meatballs, tiny, cooked in broth to keep them moist
Meats (tender varieties of lamb, veal, and beef)
Peaches, ripe, peeled
Peas, cooked
Rice
Spaghetti with meat sauce
Spaghetti squash
Sweet potato or yam, cooked and mashed or in bite-size pieces

Texture becomes of great interest at this age. Most
babies with two to four teeth are receptive to lumpier
foods. Regardless of age, babies do not need teeth to
chew soft foods; gums do an adequate job. Chewier
fruits and vegetables should be added as more teeth
erupt. It's easy to drift into the habit of serving only soft
fruits and vegetables, but it's wise to increase chewy
foods gradually as your baby's chewing ability develops.

Avoid highly acidic, uncooked fruits (such as oranges,
tangerines, and pineapple) for the under-one set.
Consider rinsing off large-curd cottage cheese in a
colander to make pieces less slippery to pick up.

Finger Foods for Babies One Year and Older

Vegetables, in Bite-Size Pieces

Asparagus tips, cooked and sliced
Broccoli florets, cooked
Carrots, soft-cooked or grated
Cauliflower, cooked
Cherry tomatoes, peeled and quartered
French fries
Green beans, cooked
Lettuce, shredded
Mushrooms, cooked
Pickle spears
Tomatoes, peeled

Fruit, in Bite-Size Pieces

Apples, peeled
Bananas, whole or cut into sections
Blueberries
Cantaloupe
Dried fruits (though avoid raisins for a while)
Grapes, halved or quartered for young toddlers
Mandarin oranges, canned, rinsed
Mango
Navel oranges, peeled, sectioned, membrane removed
Papaya
Peaches, peeled
Pears, peeled
Strawberries, halved
Sweet cherries, pitted and halved or quartered
Watermelon, pitted

Hint: A toddler who won't touch fresh fruit may love dried fruits. Soaking them in water can make them softer and easier to eat. Coating banana pieces with crushed dry cereal makes them less slippery for small fingers.

Calcium-Rich Foods, in Bite-Size Pieces

Cottage cheese (with fresh or canned fruit for interest)
Feta cheese
Grated or shredded cheese
Small squares of soft cheese such as American, Gouda, or mozzarella
Ricotta cheese, in small lumps
Yogurt (may be served semi-frozen)
Vanilla ice cream

Yogurt

Yogurt is a good baby food. It's creamy and easily digestible after your baby is ten months old. Yogurt with active cultures is healthy for the digestive tract and is lower in lactose.

Start with plain or vanilla whole-milk yogurt. It can be used as a base for fruits (such as mashed banana) or cereals, or even the fruits from baby food jars. Avoid fancy flavors and textured varieties for now. (Yogurt can also be used instead of sour cream or buttermilk for your other cooking.)

Protein Foods, in Bite-Size Pieces

Bacon, crisp*
Baked beans
Beef jerky*
Chicken or beef liver (should be served only occasionally)
Chicken or turkey
Deviled eggs made with mayonnaise
Dried beans, cooked
Frankfurters*
Ham*
Hamburger
Hard-cooked eggs
Lamb chops (with a bone that has no sharp points)
Luncheon meats*
Meatballs
Roasts, tender cuts
Sausage*
Spareribs, well-cooked, little sauce
Tofu, firm
Tuna fish
Turkey, ground and cooked like hamburger
Veal

*These meats contain sodium nitrites that act as a pre-
servative and coloring agent. They should be served in
moderation. Some experts question the nutritional safety
of nitrites, though amounts used in preservation have
declined over the years. Of even greater concern is the
large amount of fat and cholesterol these foods add to a
child's diet. Foods high in naturally occurring nitrates are
spinach, beets, and collard and turnip greens, which
should be eaten in limited amounts.

Hog Dog Hint

Since hot dogs have been the most common cause
of food-related choking among children younger
than two years of age, monitor your child's consumption of them carefully. Better yet, slice a hot
dog lengthwise (not in coin-shaped slices), and
slice the halves lengthwise again before serving
alone or on a bun.

Grains, in Bite-Size Pieces

Arrowroot cookies
Bagels and cream cheese
Biscuits
Bran muffins (slightly frozen for fewer crumbs)
Cereals, unsweetened, cold (dry or with milk or yogurt)
Cereals, hot (regular or instant)
Graham crackers
Oyster crackers
Pasta, cooked (in a variety of colors and shapes)
Pretzel rods, small (minus excess salt)
Saltines
Sandwiches, cut or broken into small pieces
Spaghetti, cooked, cut into small pieces
Toast, lightly buttered, cut into small pieces
Triscuits or other whole-grain crackers
Waffles
Zwieback

Pasta is a great favorite with tots. There's a wide variety to choose from today. The penne (tube) variety or the bow ties are easier to eat than long strands of spaghetti. However, it's easy to make long strands of spaghetti more toddler friendly by crisscrossing a bowl of spaghetti with a pizza cutter to make smaller strands. A child who disdains ground meat or spinach may devour it when it's inside a ravioli square.

Avoid ready-to-eat cereals that are sugar frosted, honey coated, or chocolate flavored. They add unnecessary sugar to your child's diet and help create a sweet tooth.

For the Determined Self-Feeder

While some little ones prefer the royal treatment of being fed, others prefer the independent route. Needless to say, encourage the latter. Here are some ways you can do this:

- Offer potatoes mashed. They adhere more easily to utensils.
- Serve a half banana (not frozen) on a wooden Popsicle stick or small plastic spoon.
- Mix dry cereal with yogurt or applesauce to make it easier to pick up with a spoon.
- Serve finger foods in a paper lunch bag. Pulling edibles out of the bag turns mealtime into a game.
- Pile food right on the highchair tray. Forget serving dishes, as they may prove to be a distraction.
- Serve puréed meats on whole-wheat toast cut into small servings like canapés.

As your child's ability to use a spoon improves, so should the variety of bowl-type foods you serve. Be patient and try not to let the mess dissuade you from letting your child continue to practice. Using a plastic mug with handles as a bowl can make self-serving easier for your child.

Teething

This early-life passage may be quiet or traumatic. Try serving slightly stale, cold, or frozen bagels; a frozen banana on a Popsicle stick; the hard core of a pineapple; or a frozen food cube on a stick. Cold washcloths are good nonfood teethers. You can offer an ice cube served in a washcloth and held in place with a secure string or rubber band. Chilled pacifiers, teething rings, or even damp washcloths can be soothing, too. Some parents prefer toothbrushes, while others offer rubber toys from pet stores.

Recipes for Teething Biscuits and Crackers

You can harden almost any bread by baking it at a very low temperature (150°F–200°F) for 15–20 minutes. Your baby will enjoy teething on a variety of hardened breads such as whole wheat, rye, or pita cut into strips. You may also try some of the following for economy and nutrition.

Eggless Teethers

1 cup instant baby cereal
1 cup flour (white, wheat, or a combination)
1 cup fruit juice

Combine and stir ingredients. If you have time, chill dough in the refrigerator. Roll out between sheets of lightly floured wax paper to about ½-inch thickness. Cut into round shapes using the top of a juice glass or a round cookie cutter. Place on a lightly greased baking sheet or one covered with parchment paper. Bake at 350°F for 40 minutes (or more) until hard.

Downright Durable Teethers

2 eggs
1 cup sugar
1 teaspoon almond or vanilla flavoring (optional)
1½–2½ cups flour (white, wheat, or a combination)

Beat eggs in a bowl and add sugar and flavoring. Mix until creamy. Gradually add enough flour to make a stiff dough. Roll out between sheets of lightly floured wax paper to about ½-inch thickness. Cut into round shapes using the top of a juice glass or a round cookie cutter. Place on a lightly greased baking sheet or one covered with parchment paper. Bake at 325°F until lightly browned and hard (about 1 hour).

Oh Baby Biscuits

1 cup baby cereal
1 cup flour (white, wheat, or a combination)
2 tablespoons cooking oil
3 egg yolks
1 4-ounce jar (or 2 packs strained) baby bananas or applesauce

Combine and stir ingredients. Roll out between sheets of lightly floured wax paper to about ½-inch thickness. Cut into round shapes using the top of a juice glass or a round cookie cutter. Place on a lightly greased baking sheet or one covered with parchment paper. Bake at 325°F until lightly browned and hard (about 1 hour).

Variation for any of the above: Roll out balls of dough into thick "logs" and bake until hard.

Banana Bread Sticks

¼ cup brown sugar
½ cup vegetable oil
2 eggs
1 cup banana, mashed
1¾ cup flour (white, whole wheat, or a combination)
2 teaspoons baking powder
½ teaspoon baking soda

Combine ingredients and stir only until smooth. Pour into a greased loaf pan. Bake at 350°F for about 1 hour or until firmly set. Cool, remove from pan, and cut into sticks. Spread sticks out on a baking sheet and bake at

150°F for 1 hour (or longer) until the sticks are hard and crunchy. Store in a tightly covered container.

Oatmeal Crackers

3 cups oatmeal, uncooked
1 cup wheat germ
2 cups flour (white, whole wheat, or a combination)
3 tablespoons sugar
¾ cup vegetable oil
1 cup water

Combine ingredients and roll onto two baking sheets. Cut into squares. Bake at 300°F for 30 minutes or until crisp. Be sure to roll thin and bake well.

Homemade Graham Crackers

1 cup flour (graham or whole wheat)
1 cup unbleached flour
1 teaspoon baking powder
¼ cup butter or margarine
½ cup sugar
¼ cup milk

Combine flours and baking powder. Cut in butter or margarine until consistency of cornmeal. Stir in sugar. Add milk to make a stiff dough. Roll out on floured surface to ¼-inch thickness. Cut into squares. Prick with a fork. Brush with milk. Bake at 400°F on an ungreased baking sheet for 18 minutes or until golden brown. If rolled thicker, these crackers can be used as teething biscuits or in Quick Graham Cracker Dessert (page 44).

Some Pass-Along Ideas

- Recycle baby food jars to use in your tool box, for rock collections, for freezing small quantities of food, for holding paints in a muffin tin, as a small bank, as spice jars, and as decorated party favors filled with treats.

- A plastic container filled with baby food jar tops provides great fun for an eight-to-twelve-month-old.

- When your child reaches the age when he or she doesn't want foods touching each other on a plate, try compartmentalized plates or molded ice cube trays.

- Nonskid appliqués or strips made for the bathtub can also prevent baby from sliding down in the highchair seat. Carry a square of nonskid webbed shelf liner in your diaper bag for restaurant highchairs.

- If you can spare a bottom drawer in your kitchen, turn it into a toy drawer. It's handy for cleanups and quick distractions!

- If your child objects to a regular bib, a colorful bandanna will do the job for your "cowboy" or "cowgirl."

- Turn a handled plastic bag into a disposable food or art bib. Cut across the bottom and up one side between the two handles. Use the handle holes for armholes.

- An egg carton can serve as a good organizer for a pebble or shell collection.

- Turn an old set of kitchen canisters into decorative supply holders next to your changing table.

- Use a straw to let children sip cooled soup.

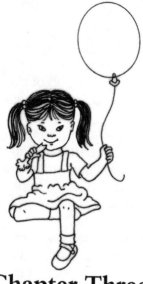

Chapter Three
Toddler Meals

With your toddler now on table foods, you'll probably notice that your meals are more often geared toward what your child will eat than what *you'd* like to eat. Save your gourmet delights for a few more years.

Although it may seem as if your child is growing like a weed, the truth is that he or she isn't growing nearly as quickly as during the first year (when birth weight triples and height nearly doubles). In general, growth rates slow down between eighteen and thirty-six months of age. That's why toddlers' calorie needs temporarily *decrease*—and why some are such finicky eaters. They simply aren't as hungry as they were as babies.

Don't let a finicky eater or a child on a food jag throw you into a tailspin. Your goal isn't to *get* your child to eat—just to *let* your child eat. Hunger will out! Just be sure that what's eaten isn't devoid of nutrients (for example, don't let your child fill up on soda pop) and don't worry about frequent snacks. Begin to look at them as minimeals.

Children have been known to survive on only peanut-but-ter-and-jelly sandwiches (or whatever) for extended peri-ods of time. And never worry about one day's intake—or lack of intake. Small children need only a little meat or other protein to fulfill the daily recommended two ounces of protein. This is the equivalent of one chicken leg, one slice of luncheon meat, or ½ cup of cooked dry beans.

Protein can be served in less obvious ways, too. Popovers (made with eggs and milk) or French Toast or Cottage-Cheese Pancakes (page 69) are finger-friendly, high-protein meals. Quesadillas (cheese melted in a microwave on rolled-up flour tortillas) are another form of a grilled cheese sandwich. Egg drop soup can be made by pouring and quickly stirring a beaten egg into boiling chicken broth.

If you're simply out of ideas, you may want to consider some of the following. Try serving them on extra-thin sliced bread.

Lunch

Participation can be a great motivator. Playing "make your own lunch" (or sandwich) often gets children to eat up their food. Have your child help you cut green onions, parsley, lettuce, cheese slices, fruit, and similar foods by using a scissors instead of a knife. Using scissors helps develop coordination and keeps kids busy for a *long* time.

Fill an empty ice cube tray with finger foods such as fresh strawberries, cheese cubes, luncheon meat, hard-cooked egg wedges, and carrot sticks. Do this early in the day, cover, and refrigerate until serving time when it will provide an interesting treat for your hard-to-please toddler.

Lunch Ideas

Deviled Ham: Spread on graham crackers or whole-wheat bread.

Cream Cheese: Spread on graham crackers. Very popular.

Egg Salad: Add mayonnaise for desired consistency. You may also wish to add finely chopped or grated celery.

Bagel Pizza: Top a bagel (or English muffin) with spaghetti sauce and shredded cheese, and broil.

Tuna Salad: Mash tuna with a fork or put it in a blender, depending on desired consistency. Mix with mayonnaise.

Lunch in a Cone: Serve tuna salad, egg salad, yogurt, or cottage cheese in a flat-bottom ice-cream cone for a different kind of "container."

Full of Baloney: Fill slices of baloney with cottage cheese, or spread with cream cheese and roll up. Secure with a toothpick.

Chicken Salad: Mix cubes of chicken with mayonnaise, finely chopped celery, and grated carrot.

Triangle Sandwiches: Spread whole-wheat bread with raspberry jam and top with thin slices of banana. Cut sandwich diagonally into fourths to make triangles.

Cottage-Cheese Salad: Combine 1 can crushed pineapple, 1 cup cottage cheese, 1 cup or so of Dream Whip, and a 3-ounce package of lime Jell-O (partially jelled) mixed according to package directions. Set gelatin more quickly by substituting 1 cup ice cubes for 1 cup cold water. (If you don't have time to prepare the Jell-O, just sprinkle a little powder from the Jell-O envelope for color and flavor.)

Cottage-Cheese Quickie: Combine a mashed kiwi (peeled) and half a banana with 1 cup cottage cheese.

French Toast: After beating eggs, use orange juice or condensed soup instead of milk with mixture.

Leftover-Meat Sandwiches: Blend about ¾ cup cubed meat, 1 hard-cooked egg, 1 tablespoon butter, and 1 tablespoon milk to make a paste. Keep in an airtight container in the refrigerator. (Puréed meat from baby food jars can also be used as a sandwich spread.)

Grilled Cheese Sandwich: Place 1–2 pieces of American cheese between 2 slices of bread. Brown on both sides in 1 tablespoon of butter in a skillet.

Deviled Eggs: Add a face by using raisins for eyes, nose, and mouth.

Other Appealing Lunch Ideas

Peanut butter is a staple in most homes with young children. Purchase brands in the refrigerated section of your grocery store, or buy ones labeled "natural" where the oil has risen to the top, since the hydrogenated oil in the shelf-stable varieties is less healthy. Check the labels regarding ingredients on shelf-stable brands, too.

A few additions to common spreads can make sandwiches more interesting and nutritious.

Peanut Butter:
- With ground raisins mixed with fruit juice
- With grated raw carrots
- Topped with applesauce
- And banana slices
- And cream cheese, blended with 2 tablespoons orange juice or honey

Cream Cheese with:
- Jelly
- Ground raisins
- Peeled and finely chopped (or grated) cucumber
- Chopped egg, cheese, and bacon
- Cottage cheese and grated pineapple
- Cottage cheese topped with sliced hard-cooked egg

Keep your sliced bread in the freezer to keep it from tearing when peanut butter or cream cheese is spread on it. You'll find that sliced bread thaws in only a few minutes, so work quickly.

Pancakes are another excellent "bread" for sandwich spreads. Make (and freeze) extras the next time you're having them, or buy the frozen variety. After applying a spread, pop them in the microwave for 30–45 seconds before serving.

Homemade Alphabet Soup

1 teaspoon alphabet noodles
2 teaspoons instant tapioca
⅔ cup vegetable broth
dash of salt
dot of butter

Cook over high heat for 3 minutes, stirring constantly. Remove from heat. Stir in a dash of salt and a dot of butter.

Dinner

One of dinnertime's biggest problems is that your child's stomach is inevitably a half hour to an hour ahead of your meal schedule. You can feed your child early and avoid the next hour's headache. If you're determined to have the whole family eat together, offer a salad, side dish, or carrot as an appetizer. Sugarless gum or bubble gum may work to delay a hungry older child. (Don't give chewing gum, which is a choking hazard, to a child younger than four years old.)

For younger toddlers who are ready to eat corn-on-the-cob but not digest the hulls, slice off the tops of the kernels, or slice down the middles of each row of kernels, so the corn can be sucked out.

And do you find that your child simply can't sit still during a meal? He or she must stand, bounce, climb, kick the table, go to the toilet, and generally drive you bananas. We can offer no remedy—only sympathy, for you're not alone. (We probably performed these same foul deeds as kids ourselves.)

Hint: An ice cube can bring many cooked foods to an edible temperature quickly. Toddlers are not in favor of foods hot from the stove or oven.

Dinner Ideas

Tiny Meatballs: Add beaten eggs, oatmeal or wheat germ, and grated cheese.

Meat Loafies: Add ingredients above, but cook in a muffin tin. (Freezes well in this form. Reheat on a baking sheet in oven or toaster oven.)

Macaroni and Cheese: Serve your combo or the grocer's. An all-time favorite.

Chicken Livers: Sauté in butter until tender and cut into pieces. Or wrap in bacon and broil.

Boned Fish: Use only fish that's quite flaky, such as cod. Always check carefully for bones.

Corned Beef Hash: Place in a frying pan. Make a depression with the back of a spoon and break an egg into it. Cover and heat until egg is firm. Messy with fingers, but not bad with a spoon.

Pineapple Franks: Split frankfurters lengthwise and fill with drained pineapple. Broil 5–10 minutes. Older toddlers enjoy these.

Omelets: Cook beaten eggs plain or with such additions as onions, green pepper, cheese, or wheat germ as large pancakes rather than scrambled. It's much easier and neater for a child to eat omelets broken into pieces.

Tuna Burgers

1 7-ounce can tuna, drained
2 tablespoons onion, chopped

2 tablespoons pickle, chopped
¼ cup mayonnaise
hamburger buns
slice of cheese, optional

Combine first four ingredients. Split and toast hamburger buns. Spread bottom half with tuna mixture. Top with a slice of cheese and broil for 4 minutes or until cheese melts. Add bun tops.

Tuna Patties

⅔ cup Grape-Nuts cereal
½ cup milk
1 cup onion, finely chopped
2 tablespoons butter or margarine
2 7-ounce cans tuna, drained
2 eggs, slightly beaten
1 teaspoon lemon juice

Add cereal to milk; set aside. Sauté onions in 1 table-spoon butter or margarine until tender but not browned. Add tuna, eggs, onions, and lemon juice to cereal mixture. Blend thoroughly. Makes 12 patties. Brown on both sides in 1 tablespoon butter or margarine.

Salmon Soufflé

1 16-ounce can boneless, skinless salmon
1 7¾-ounce can evaporated milk
3 tablespoons butter
3 tablespoons flour
½ teaspoon dry mustard
4 eggs, separated
paprika, optional

Drain salmon liquid into 8-ounce measuring cup and add enough milk to make 1 cup. In saucepan, melt butter and blend in flour and dry mustard. Gradually add milk and cook, stirring until thickened. Remove from heat. Stir in beaten egg yolks and flaked salmon; cool. Beat egg whites until stiff and fold into mixture. Pour into buttered 2-quart soufflé or casserole dish and bake at 350°F for 45–50 minutes. Dust with paprika.

Loafer's Loaf

1 pound ground beef
1¼ cup uncooked old fashioned (not instant) oatmeal
¼ cup minced onion
¼ cup American cheese, grated
½ teaspoon celery salt
1 cup milk
⅔ cup tomatoes, chopped
1 egg, beaten

Combine all ingredients. Pack into greased loaf pan. Bake at 350°F for 1 hour and 10 minutes.

Sloppy Poodles

1 pound lean ground beef
2 tablespoons flour
1 10-ounce can condensed French onion soup
6 hot dog (or hamburger) buns

Brown meat in large skillet and drain off excess fat. Sprinkle flour over meat and stir until flour disappears. Add can of undiluted soup. Simmer for a few minutes until mixture thickens and becomes hot. Serve on buns. (Hot dog buns are easier for kids to hold than hamburger buns.)

South-of-the-Border Casserole

1 15-ounce can chili
1 12- or 17-ounce can whole-kernel corn
1 8-ounce package grated cheese
1–2 cups baked tortilla chips

Combine chili and corn in an oven or microwave-safe dish. Add grated cheese and then crumble chips. Press them down gently part way into the mixture. Bake in a 350°F oven for 20 minutes or 5–8 minutes in a microwave.

Simple Soufflé

¼ cup butter or margarine, melted
¼ cup flour
1 cup milk
1 cup cheddar, Swiss, or mozzarella cheese, shredded (optional)
4 eggs
¼ teaspoon cream of tartar

Melt butter. Stir in flour. Cook over medium heat until bubbly. Add milk gradually and stir constantly until smooth and thickened. Add cheese if you're using it. Beat 2 egg yolks until smooth. Blend a little of the hot mixture into the yolk mixture. Return yolk mixture to saucepan and blend. Remove from heat. Pour into 1½-quart casserole. Beat 4 egg whites until stiff (not dry) along with cream of tartar. Fold into casserole dish. Bake at 350°F for 30–40 minutes. Delicious even when it falls.

Simpler Soufflé

1 10-ounce can condensed cheddar-cheese soup
6 eggs, yolks and whites whipped separately

Combine beaten egg yolks and cheese soup in a casserole dish. Fold in egg whites. Bake at 400°F for 40 minutes or until done.

Orange Chicken

2 chicken legs and thighs
2 tablespoons butter, melted
½ cup orange juice
poultry seasoning

Place chicken in small baking dish. Mix melted butter with orange juice. Pour over chicken. Sprinkle with poultry seasoning. Bake 15 minutes at 350°F. Turn and baste with juice mixture. Broil for 15 minutes or until chicken skin is crisp.

Chicken Quiche

½ cup chicken, cooked and diced
1 9-inch pie shell, unbaked
1½ cups Swiss cheese, shredded
3 eggs, slightly beaten
1½ cups milk
2 tablespoons Parmesan cheese, grated

Place chicken in pie shell and add Swiss cheese. Combine eggs and milk. Pour over cheese. Sprinkle on Parmesan cheese. Bake at 375°F for 30–35 minutes or until a knife inserted into the center comes out clean. Let stand 10 minutes before serving.

Veggies

"If it's green, it must be yucky" is a philosophy you might run into—like a stone wall. Just increase the variety of fruits in your child's menu until your child's taste tolerance widens. Some parents like to require their children to eat the same number of bites of vegetables as their individual ages. This adds pros and cons to being the oldest or the youngest child.

One way of introducing your child to a new vegetable, such as an artichoke, is by *not* serving it. "Adult only" food often becomes more desirable when treated as forbidden fruit. You can *perhaps* let your child have a taste from your plate. Graduating to "adult" foods makes children feel more grown-up and at the very least saves you from throwing out or arguing over some tasty part of your meal.

Keep in mind that canned vegetables are generally high in salt. Look for canned choices that offer "low sodium."

Tips for Getting Your Child to Eat Vegetables

- Use up any leftover (cooked) yellow or white vegetable by mashing it, mixing it with an egg, and cooking it like a pancake or baking it in a muffin tin.
- Sprinkle shredded cheese over each spoonful of cooked vegetables. Or better yet, let your little cheese lover do the job!
- Purée steamed vegetables and add to a simmering broth for a creamy soup.
- Have you tried spaghetti squash? This yellow, oval squash can be cooked whole in the microwave until soft. Cut it in half, remove the seeds, then use a fork to remove the flesh. It comes up like spaghetti strands. Serve with butter, margarine, a little olive oil, or spaghetti sauce. A good early finger food.
- Desperate? Try green noodles. They're made with spinach.
- Add moderate amounts of finely chopped vegetables to a cheese omelet.
- Be creative. Artistic food ideas often inspire young eaters. Use greens (broccoli, peas, and lettuce) as treetops and pretzels as trunks. Half of a cherry tomato can be the center of a sun or a clown's nose. Shredded carrot can look like hair. Creating fun names for foods can also be effective.
- Hide puréed vegetables (in moderate amounts) in meat loaf and spaghetti sauce. Hide a little purée under melted cheese on pizza, or mix it with mashed potatoes (especially effective with a little cauliflower). You might even want to try this with hamburgers. Experiment. Do it gradually.
- Mash some canned black beans into meat used for hamburger or meatballs.
- If you're serving dessert, try one made with a vegetable, like pumpkin pie or carrot cake.
- Make sweet-potato chips. Place 12 thin, unpeeled, sweet potato circle slices on a microwave rack. Sprinkle with cinnamon sugar and microwave 4–5

minutes until dry. Rotate during cooking. Let cool before eating.

Honeyed Carrots

3 tablespoons butter or margarine
4 cups carrots, sliced
3 tablespoons orange juice
¼ teaspoon ginger
4 tablespoons honey

Combine all ingredients in a saucepan and cover. Cook over low heat for 30 minutes or until tender. Stir occasionally. Leftovers may be frozen.

Un"beet"able Gelatin

1 jar strained baby beets
cold water
1 3-ounce package strawberry Jell-O
1 cup boiling water

Chill strained beets thoroughly, then combine with cold water to make 1 cup liquid. Set aside. Dissolve Jell-O in boiling water and add liquid beet mixture. Chill until set.

Variation: Substitute cooked and puréed fresh or canned beets for baby food jar equivalent. Beets vary, depending upon the season. If not sweet enough alone, add 1 teaspoon sugar to beet mixture.

Green–Bean Bake

2 packages whole green beans, frozen
1 garlic clove, sliced (optional)
¼ teaspoon pepper (optional)
1 cup sour cream or plain yogurt
2 tablespoons butter
bread crumbs

Cook green beans with garlic following label directions. Drain. Place in baking dish. Stir pepper into sour cream and spoon over beans. Melt butter in small saucepan. Add bread crumbs and toss. Sprinkle bread crumbs over sour cream. Bake at 350°F for 20 minutes.

Raw Vegetables

Raw vegetables often meet with less resistance than cooked. If your toddler attacks the hors d'oeuvre tray when your company is starting on cocktails, then you may have discovered a fresh approach: serve raw vegetables with dip.

Good vegetable options for children include carrots, celery, cauliflower, radishes, cucumber spears, broccoli, sliced zucchini, slivers of green pepper, or mushrooms. The dip can have yogurt, sour cream, cheese, or tahini as a base.

Older toddlers are often fond of nibbling on frozen green peas straight from the freezer bag. Or try sugar snap peas—they're sweet. Often children will eat vegetables they pick from a summer garden while passing over the same item from your refrigerator.

Don't forget that, while not green, potatoes are an excellent vegetable. A baked potato, which takes only 3–4 minutes to cook in a microwave, can be a meal by itself, especially when topped with cheese, sour cream, spaghetti sauce, or anything else your child loves. And of course it can be mashed, baked twice, and, yes, even fried!

Bunny Food

Combine grated carrots with raisins. Mix with some mayonnaise or a bit of honey and lemon juice.

Pickled Carrots

For a new flavored snack, store carrot sticks in pickle jars that still have liquid in them.

Quick Desserts

Quick Graham Cracker Dessert

Crumble 1 graham cracker into a bowl. Add a teaspoon of honey and a bit of warm milk. Mash, mix, and serve.

Yogurt Sundae

Put some yogurt (frozen or not) in a dish. Add fresh fruit and pour honey over the fruit. Sprinkle with granola, nuts, or toasted wheat germ. Top with a maraschino cherry.

No-Work Dessert

Serve any fresh fruit with small, separate bowls of brown sugar and sour cream or yogurt. Dip the fruit in the brown sugar, then in the sour cream, and eat.

Chocolate Cream Cheese

1 tablespoon cream cheese
1 teaspoon milk
½ teaspoon sugar
⅛ teaspoon cocoa

Beat cream cheese with milk until smooth. Then beat in sugar and cocoa.

Apple Custard

1 apple
2 tablespoons sugar
1 egg

Wash, peel, and core apple. Slice very thin and sprinkle with sugar. Beat the egg and fold into the apples. Put these into a well-buttered baking dish. Bake at 350°F for 30 minutes.

Baked Banana

Peel firm bananas and place in a well-greased baking dish. Brush with butter and bake at 350°F for 12–15 minutes. Remove from oven. With the tip of a spoon, make a shallow groove the length of the banana and fill with honey.

Banana and Apple Whip

1 small apple
1 small banana
1 teaspoon milk
¼ teaspoon sugar

Wash, peel, and cut apple into small pieces, or grate it. Add the remaining ingredients and beat until blended. Serve immediately.

Banana Instant Pudding

2 ripe bananas, mashed
½ cup applesauce
2 tablespoons peanut butter
2 tablespoons honey

Stir ingredients until smooth, then chill. Sprinkle with cinnamon or wheat germ before serving.

Homemade Fresh-Fruit Sherbet

1¼ cups fresh fruit
1 cup sugar
2 pasteurized egg whites, beaten

Cut the fruit into small pieces and mix well with sugar. Beat egg whites stiff and fold them in. Put in a freezer tray and freeze for about 2 hours, stirring occasionally. Cover with wax paper until ready to serve.

Chocolate "Ice Cream"

½ can sweetened condensed milk
1½ tablespoons cocoa
½ cup regular milk

Combine ingredients and freeze for about 3 hours in a freezer tray.

Nutritious Frostings

Base:
2 tablespoons soft butter or margarine
¼ cup honey
1 teaspoon vanilla

Cream together. For flavorings, add the following to the base and whip until smooth. (*Don't tell your children that the frosting is nutritious or they'll decide it's yucky before trying it.*) Use on breads and muffins as well as cookies and cakes.

Fruity Frosting

2–3 tablespoons fruit juice
1 cup nonfat dry milk
grated orange or lemon rind or chopped raisins or dates

Variation: You can substitute peanut butter for the butter or margarine in the base and add whatever else appeals to your family. Be sure to include the dry milk.

Spice Frosting

2–3 tablespoons milk, buttermilk, or yogurt
1 cup nonfat dry milk
dashes of cinnamon, nutmeg, and allspice

Banana Frosting

Mash 1 banana and add to Spice Frosting.

Chocolate or Carob Frosting

2–3 tablespoons milk, yogurt, or buttermilk
¼ cup cocoa powder or carob powder
⅔ cup nonfat dry milk

More Frostings

- Sprinkle sugar and cinnamon on a cake or cookies just as you would on toast.
- Melt ½ 6-ounce package of chocolate chips and mix with ½ cup peanut butter. Spread over cookies or bars.
- Spread honey on cookies to make a good "glue" for adding candy décors, coconut, and other decorations.
- Dust confectioners' sugar on a cake or bar recipe for a completed look.
- Mix 1 tablespoon thawed orange juice concentrate with 1 cup powdered sugar to make a "dribble" frosting.

Beverages

The following beverages make good meal supplements or snacks. When your baby graduates to cow's milk at around one year of age, you should serve whole milk until your child is at least two years old. The fat in whole milk is essential for young children's growth and development.

Hint: Leftover formula can be used for cooking, baking, or even in coffee.

Yogurt Milk Shake

1 cup vanilla yogurt
1 cup orange juice
1 ripe banana

Blend.

Tropical Blend

½ cup vanilla yogurt
½ cup crushed pineapple, undrained
¼ cup orange juice
½ kiwi or banana, peeled

Blend. If too thick, add 1–3 ice cubes.

Sunny Sipper

½ cup orange juice
3 tablespoons lemon juice
1 13-ounce can evaporated milk
1 13-ounce can apricot nectar

Blend. Serve chilled.

Banana Smoothie

1½ cups milk
1 large banana
¼ teaspoon vanilla

Blend and serve at once. The banana can be one that you've peeled and frozen.

Variation: Add a tablespoon of peanut butter before blending.

Triple Shake

1 cup each of three different fruits
5 ice cubes

Blend fruits and ice cubes for a thick fruit shake. Experiment with various combinations. This is also an excellent way to use up those last pieces of ripe fruit. Or, slice them up and freeze them in a plastic bag until you're ready to use them.

Sangria Junior

To 1 small bottle of white grape juice or cranberry juice in a wide-mouth pitcher, add:

1 cup orange juice
1 cup sliced grapes (optional)
1 cup orange circles, sliced in half
1 cup strawberries, kiwis, apples, or peaches, cleaned and sliced

Serve with swizzle sticks or long forks and a straw.

Milk Eggnog

1 cup cold milk
1 pasteurized egg
¼ teaspoon vanilla
1 tablespoon honey
nonfat dry milk (optional)

Blend. Eggnog is another way of providing protein for an older toddler who frequently refuses other protein foods. Fortify with several tablespoons of nonfat dry milk if you wish.

Variation: Orange juice may be substituted for milk.

Egg Alert

Some of these drink recipes call for raw eggs, which is a good way of sneaking eggs into those children for whom *egg* means "Forget it!" Most physicians don't recommend serving whole eggs (raw or cooked) to babies under one year of age, since some infants have an allergic reaction to egg white. Use only cooked yolks for babies six to twelve months of age, and freeze the whites for later use in baking.

Because raw eggs can carry salmonella bacteria, always use pasteurized eggs in uncooked recipes that call for eggs.

Orange Delight

1–2 pasteurized eggs
⅓ cup orange juice concentrate
¼ cup nonfat dry milk
½ banana (or equivalent fruit)
¾ cup water
ice

Mix in blender. The more ice you add, the slushier the drink becomes.

Water

The preceding beverages are great snacks, but kids also need to satisfy their thirst and their bodies' need for fluids. Water is still the best (and cheapest) thirst quencher. Make drinking it an early habit. Sometimes kids need to have the appeal of water reinforced by fun containers (a biker's bottle, a canteen, or a new plastic cup). Keeping water cold also enhances its appeal.

Juices labeled "100% real fruit juice"—*not juice drinks*—are also good beverage options. Be aware that apple juice in large amounts can contribute to chronic diarrhea in young children. You may wish to water it down if you have an "apple juice only" child. Avoid sodas as a staple—especially those high in caffeine such as colas and chocolate-flavored or some fruit-fla-vored sodas. For the same reason, go easy on iced tea. Many doctors recommend waiting until your child is one year old before introducing orange juice, given its high acid content and allergy risk.

Milk

After water, your next best beverage for toddlers is whole milk. Sixteen to twenty-four ounces of milk a day is plenty for a toddler over age one. Toddlers who eat yogurt, cheese, and other dairy products can get by with less. Don't switch to low-fat or skim milk until your child is at least two years old or your doctor recommends a change. Here are some ways to improve milk's appeal, if needed.

Milk Marvels

Add one of the following to 1 cup of cold milk, and mix well in a blender:

- ½ banana, mashed or frozen
- 1 scoop fruit-flavored ice cream, sherbet, or frozen yogurt
- ½ cup frozen strawberries plus the juice, or ½ cup fresh berries plus some sweetener, if needed
- ½ cup fresh bruised berries, 1 teaspoon sugar, and 1 tablespoon lemon or orange juice
- ½ banana, 1 scoop vanilla ice cream, and 1 tablespoon chocolate syrup
- canned peaches or pears with 2 tablespoons juice from can and 1 scoop vanilla ice cream

To a mug of hot cocoa and milk, add a spoonful of creamy peanut butter and a dash of whipped cream.

Fortified Milk

The protein value of milk can be increased by adding some nonfat dry milk to regular milk. But do so only in moderation, especially if your child already has a low fluid intake. *Never give a calcium supplement without professional advice.*

Hint: For the child who refuses milk, remember that it can be "eaten" in the form of puddings, custards, cheese, yogurt, or creamy soups.

Hints for the do-it-yourself (at last!) drinker:
- Fill a glass only about ⅓ full to limit waste when the inevitable spills occur. Provide refills when requested.
- Have your child practice drinking water from a cup while he or she is taking a bath.

51

- Cut straws down to size for the child and cup (or glass) being used.

If Your Child Can't Drink Cow's Milk

Milk intolerance is a common problem that defies the old slogan "Milk. It Does a Body Good." Not every body. Actually, the majority of the world's population can't tolerate cow's milk. Those most able to do so are of Western European descent, and even among this group, a significant percentage (20%–25%) can't tolerate milk. Symptoms such as abdominal pain, bloating, gas, diarrhea, or nausea may be related to the ingestion of cow's milk.

This intolerance, referred to as "lactose intolerance," results from an inability to digest the natural sugar in milk. An enzyme (lactase) in the intestinal lining breaks down lactose (milk sugar) into simple, digestible sugars. When lactase is completely absent (a rare condition) or present in low concentrations (which is more common), consumption of milk products may cause discomfort. In a young child, an intestinal infection can cause temporary reduction of lactase. This is one reason why doctors eliminate milk when a child has diarrhea.

The amount of milk tolerable to those with lactose intolerance varies with the level of lactase in the intestine. For example, some people who can't digest moderate amounts of milk can tolerate yogurt or aged cheeses.

When reading food, vitamin, and medication labels, watch for the words milk (condensed, evaporated, fresh, whole, skim), buttermilk, sweet or sour cream, malted milk, lactose, nonfat dry milk solids, curds, whey, margarine, butter, sodium caseinate, casein, and lactalbumin. (The last three are additives made from the protein of cow's milk and are permissible for those who cannot tolerate lactose—but not for those who are allergic to milk.)

Cooking Milk-Free

In cooking, you can often substitute another liquid for milk. When a recipe calls for milk, try soymilk. Use unflavored, unsweetened, vitamin-enriched, full-fat soymilk for best results and maximun nutrition. For cream, you can substitute unflavored soymilk creamer. If someone in your family has a soy allergy, try water, chicken stock, beef stock, or fruit juices. Orange juice and apple juice—even 7-UP—work nicely in many recipes for baked products. With a bit of experimenting, you'll find substitutes that work for you.

Or maybe you've discovered Lactaid Milk (lactose-free) or Lactaid Dietary Supplements, which help restore the enzyme in the body that makes dairy foods more digestible. For a free sample or information, call 800-LACTAID or visit www.lactaid.com. Another product on the market is Land O Lakes Dairy Ease (www.dairyease.com).

Puddle Cake

This classic dessert is also milk-free.

1½ cups flour (white or half-white-half-whole-wheat)
1 cup sugar
1 teaspoon baking soda
3 tablespoons cocoa or carob powder
1 teaspoon vanilla
1 teaspoon vinegar
6 tablespoons vegetable oil
1 cup water

Sift flour, sugar, soda, and cocoa into an ungreased 8-by-10-inch cake pan. With a mixing spoon, make three holes in the dry mixture. Place vanilla in the first hole, vinegar in the second, and oil in the third. Pour water over all and stir with a fork to moisten dry ingredients. Do not beat. Bake at 350°F for 35 minutes.

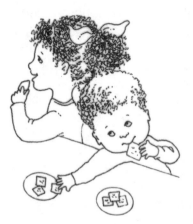

Chapter Four
Snacks

Snacking is a way of life in most American households. It need not be a dirty word—nor need it involve junk food! Junky snacks push the nutritious foods out of kids' diets, contribute to tooth decay, and add pounds. However, nutritious snacks should be considered part of your child's overall nutrition for the day.

Kids snack on what's handy. Having wholesome snacks on hand—store-bought or homemade—is part of a parent's job. Fruits and vegetables are the most obvious nutritious snack foods, plus most of the finger foods listed in previous chapters.

Crackers are lower in sugar than cookies. Many are now available in reduced-salt versions. And don't forget whole-grain toast. Toast can be made more interesting by buttering it lightly or sprinkling it with a little cinnamon and sugar, or Parmesan cheese, before cutting it with a cookie cutter. (You can use one shape at a time for a theme, such as a fish-shaped cookie cutter for a "fishy" snack, or different shapes.) Place shapes on a baking sheet and toast lightly in an oven at 350°F.

Spread mashed bananas (or any other favored spread) on mini rice cakes or pita bread for a healthy snack.

Raisins and other dried fruits have fallen from favor in the dental community because they consist of sugars (albeit natural) that stick between children's teeth and promote tooth decay. Consider moving dried fruits from snack time to the main mealtime.

And don't rule out cold, cooked pastas. Elbow macaroni by itself or served with grated cheese makes a good snack food.

Finger Jell-O

> 2 envelopes unflavored gelatin
> 2½ cups water
> 1 6-ounce package (or 2 3-ounce packages) Jell-O

It disappears before your very eyes! Dissolve unflavored gelatin in 1 cup cold water. Set aside. In a saucepan, bring 1 cup water to a boil and add Jell-O. Bring to a boil again, then remove from heat. Add gelatin mixture. Stir and add ½ cup cold water. Pour into a lightly greased pan and refrigerate until firm (about 2 hours). Cut into squares (or use a cookie cutter) and store in an airtight container in the refrigerator.

Variation: You can avoid using commercial Jell-O by combining 3 envelopes of unflavored gelatin with 1 12-ounce can of frozen juice concentrate and 12 ounces of water. Soften the gelatin in the thawed juice and bring the water to a boil. Add juice-and-gelatin mixture to the boiling water and stir until gelatin dissolves. If the juice needs extra sweetening, add it here. Follow directions for chilling as indicated above.

Jell-O Pizza

Mix above recipe for Finger Jell-O using lemon- or orange-flavored gelatin. Pour in just enough to fill a lightly greased pizza pan to the edges, and chill in refrigerator until firm. (Chill balance of Jell-O in a second pizza pan or another container.) Spread vanilla yogurt or whipped cream lightly on the firm Jell-O. Sprinkle sliced fruits (such as kiwis, bananas, or strawberries) on top. Cut into wedges and serve.

Apples in Hand

Peel (optional) and core a whole apple. Mix peanut butter with one of the following: raisins, wheat germ, or granola. Stuff this mixture into the hole of the cored apple. Slice in half to serve. Or stick the apple half on a Popsicle stick. It's both novel and neat that way.

Stuffed Celery

Stuff celery sticks with cream cheese or peanut butter. Raisins may be added on top of the spread. Depending on the age and chewing ability of the child, you may want to remove the strands from the celery.

Turn a stuffed celery stick into a "racing car" by pushing a toothpick through each end of the celery piece and attaching a single grape to each end of the toothpicks for "wheels." *But make sure your child doesn't eat the toothpicks*!

Grinder Snacks

Grind figs, dates, and raisins in equal amounts. (Nutmeats, too, if you wish.) Add a small amount of lemon juice to a cup of graham cracker crumbs. Make small balls out of your ground mixture and roll in crumbs for coating. (Your baby food grinder can come in handy here.)

Peanut-Butter Roll-Ups

4 slices bread
1 container peanut butter
honey or jam (optional)

Trim crusts from bread slices. Place slices on a hard surface and use a rolling pin to roll them flat. Spread a thin

57

layer of peanut butter onto each slice of flattened bread. Spread jam or drizzle honey onto peanut butter. Roll up each slice of bread jellyroll style. Slice roll-ups into one-inch pieces and secure with toothpicks.

Peanut–Butter Balls

½ cup peanut butter
3½ tablespoons nonfat dry milk
bit of honey
optional: raisins, nuts, coconut, wheat germ, sunflower seeds,
*   and brown sugar*

Combine ingredients, roll into balls, and store in refrigerator.

Goodie Balls

½ cup peanut butter
½ cup honey
½ cup instant cocoa or carob powder
1 cup peanuts or soy nuts, chopped
½ cup sunflower seeds
1 cup toasted wheat germ
dry coconut flakes

Combine first six ingredients. Roll into balls and roll in coconut. Refrigerate if using a refrigerated brand of peanut butter, which is preferable.

Chocolate Peanut–Butter Sticks

8 ounces semisweet chocolate
6 tablespoons peanut butter
1 teaspoon vanilla
1 cup toasted wheat germ

Melt chocolate and blend with peanut butter and vanilla. Stir in wheat germ. Press into a buttered 8-by-8-inch pan and chill until firm. Cut into bars and store in a container in the refrigerator.

Cheesy Wheats

½ cup butter or margarine
1 cup cheese, shredded
4 cups Spoon Size Shredded Wheat

Melt butter or margarine in a large saucepan. Add cheese. When cheese begins to melt, add Shredded Wheat. Toss to coat well. Refrigerate if not to be eaten within an hour or two. (This recipe can be easily adapted for a microwave.)

Cereal Sticks

½ cup butter or margarine
1 cup sugar
2 eggs
1 teaspoon vanilla
2½ cups flour (white, whole wheat, or a combination)
¼ teaspoon baking soda
½ cup (or more) of cereal, such as Grape-Nuts, granola,
  or wheat germ

Blend first six ingredients plus ¼ cup cereal. If dough is too soft, add more flour. Roll small piece of dough into a stick, then roll the stick in the extra cereal to coat. (Employ anyone in your family who's experienced with play dough.) Place on a lightly greased baking sheet and bake at 400°F for 8 minutes or until slightly browned.

Uncandy Bars

1 loaf of bread (white, whole wheat, or other)
1 package peanuts, chopped
¼ cup toasted wheat germ (optional)
1 cup peanut butter
peanut oil

Trim crust from bread and cut bread slices in half. Put bread and crusts on a baking sheet in the oven

overnight, until dry, or place in a 150°F oven for ½ hour
or until dry. Put only the dried crusts in a blender until
finely crumbed. Combine crumbs with chopped nuts.
Add wheat germ, if desired. Thin the peanut butter with
oil. Spread or dip the bread slices in the peanut butter,
then roll them in the nut-and-crumb mixture. Dry them on
a baking sheet. Store in an airtight container. No need to
refrigerate if you're using shelf-stable peanut butter.

Variation: If candy isn't "candy" to you without chocolate,
add 1 tablespoon instant cocoa to the thinned peanut butter.

Oatmeal Bars

¾ cup brown sugar
½ cup butter or margarine
dash of baking soda
2 cups oatmeal, uncooked

Boil sugar, butter or margarine, and baking soda. Add
oatmeal. Blend. Spread mixture in a well-greased 8-by-8-
inch pan and bake at 350°F for 10 minutes. Cut into bars
while warm.

Bite-of-Apple Cookies

½ cup margarine
1 cup brown sugar
2 eggs
1½ cups flour
½ cup oatmeal, uncooked
2 teaspoons baking soda
½ teaspoon cinnamon
¾ cup wheat germ
1 cup apples, peeled, cored, and finely chopped

Cream margarine, sugar, and eggs. Mix dry ingredients
and combine with creamed mixture. Add apples. Drop
spoonfuls onto a greased baking sheet. Bake at 350°F
for 10–15 minutes.

Super Cookies

1½ cups old-fashioned (not instant) oatmeal, uncooked
  (or Familia Swiss Muesli)
½ cup nonfat dry milk
½ cup wheat germ
¾ cup sugar (or ½ cup honey)
1 teaspoon cinnamon
⅓ teaspoon cloves
½ cup butter, melted, or vegetable oil
2 eggs, beaten

Mix dry ingredients. Add melted butter or vegetable oil and beaten eggs. Spoon onto greased baking sheet. Bake at 350°F for 12–15 minutes.

Nutritious Brownies

¼ cup vegetable oil
1 tablespoon molasses
1 cup brown sugar
2 teaspoons vanilla
2 eggs
½ cup pecans or walnuts, broken
1 cup wheat germ
⅔ cup nonfat dry milk
½ teaspoon baking powder
¼ cup dry cocoa or 2 squares unsweetened baking chocolate

Mix the first seven ingredients. (If using squares of chocolate, melt in a double boiler and add here.) Sift the dry milk, baking powder, and cocoa through a sieve into the other ingredients and stir well. Spread in a heavily greased 8-by-8-inch pan and bake at 350°F for approximately 30 minutes. Turn out of pan immediately and cut into bars while still warm.

Fruit Roll

Use apples, peaches, pears, nectarines, or canned pumpkin to make this yummy dried "candy." The fruit can be the "too hard to eat" variety or the "too ripe" or "last piece" variety. It may even be well-drained canned fruit.

Mash or purée the fruit. Two methods work well:

Blender method: Peel and core fruit, blend until smooth, and cook for 5 minutes in a saucepan over medium heat.

Freeze-defrost method: Peel and core fruit in advance, then wrap and freeze. Remove from freezer an hour before using so fruit can begin to defrost. Cook in a saucepan, mashing with a fork as you go, for 5–10 minutes. If the fruit is very watery, drain it.

While cooking, add 1 teaspoon honey for each piece of fruit you're using. (Cook different fruits separately, though you can cook one piece or a dozen of the same type at once.)

Lay out clear plastic wrap (or cut open small plastic bags) on a baking sheet or broiling tray. Use one piece of plastic for each piece of fruit you've cooked. Spoon mixture onto the wrap, staying away from its edge. Spread as thin as possible. Spread another piece of plastic wrap over the mixture and press down with a wide spatula to make evenly thin. Remove this top sheet of plastic before drying.

Turn oven to its lowest possible heat or just use the pilot light. Place tray in the oven and leave overnight (6–8 hours). The plastic wrap will not melt! If the fruit is dry by breakfast, remove from the oven. (If not, wait a while longer.) Roll up the plastic wrap (with the dried fruit) as if it were a jellyroll. Then peel and eat!

The rolls will last several months this way—if your children don't discover them, that is. If you don't understand how this should look, stop at a health-food store and ask to look at their fruit rolls. And notice the price!

Variation: Core and peel an apple. Slice it into thin rings and dry according to instructions above.

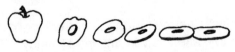

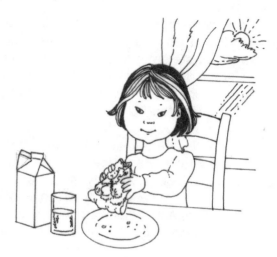

Chapter Five
Pizza for Breakfast?

It's 7:45 in the morning. Your husband needs to leave for work by 8:15, and you need to be out by 9:00. He's in the kitchen frying some eggs. You're nursing your three-month-old, and your three-year-old doesn't want fried eggs. He'd rather have leftover pizza for breakfast. Your husband says, "No, pizza isn't breakfast food. Here's a nice piece of toast with jelly." Your three-year-old rejects that, too. You finish feeding and changing the baby, and give your three-year-old some cold sugared cereal with milk and a glass of orange juice. Then you drink a cup of coffee or tea and plan to have something to eat later. Sound familiar?

No one wants to be creative at 7 AM, but breakfast is a very important meal. And it's important for you to be a good model for your kids in this area as in other aspects of your life. People who skip breakfast are more likely to eat between meals and often consume more calories in a day than people who eat breakfast. If your children see you eating a well-balanced breakfast, they'll probably develop good eating habits, too.

Part of the problem stems from our stereotyped ideas about breakfast food, as illustrated above. Maybe it's time to change our stereotypes about mealtime menus. A peanut-butter sandwich, a hunk of cheese and whole-wheat toast, or a container of yogurt are perfectly acceptable breakfast foods.

Leftovers such as pizza, hamburger, casseroles, chops, or spaghetti have traditionally been served at lunch and dinner. Why not serve them for breakfast? And save the eggs, cereal, or "breakfasty" items for lunch or dinner? You don't even have to warm up the leftovers!

The following ideas and recipes are intended to make breakfast enjoyable *and* nutritious not only for your kids, but for your entire family.

Breakfast Pizza

If you have leftover spaghetti sauce, here's a good way to use it up!

English muffins
butter or margarine
spaghetti sauce
cheese (such as mozzarella, cheddar, American, or Colby), sliced

Split muffins and toast lightly. Spread a little butter or margarine on each half and add 1–2 tablespoons of spaghetti sauce. You may also add bacon, mushrooms, or anything else that's handy. Lay a slice or two of cheese on top. Heat muffin "pizzas" in the broiler or toaster oven until the cheese is gooey (3–5 minutes).

Other nontraditional possibilities for breakfast include:
- Grilled (or ungrilled) cheese sandwiches
- Cottage cheese
- Soup and cheese
- Eggnog drinks (page 49)

Eggs

Eggs are a traditional part of the breakfast scene. Some kids really go for them while others do not. Eggs are a good dinner option, too. Here are a few ideas that might not convert the egg haters but may lure the "not so crazy about eggs" bunch!

Bull's Eye

1 slice bread
butter or margarine
1 egg

Use a 2-inch-round cookie cutter to cut out the center of the bread. Spread margarine generously on both sides of the remaining bread. Brown one side of the bread in a moderately hot, greased frying pan, and then turn over. Crack the egg into the hole in the bread and cook until the white is set and the yolk begins to thicken. You may need to cover the pan to help the egg set quickly. Lift out carefully and serve.

You may wish to use a cookie cutter shaped as a heart for Valentine's Day, a bunny for Easter, and a bell for Christmas.

Peanut-Butter Custard

1⅓ cups milk
⅓ cup nonfat dry milk
⅓ cup peanut butter
2 eggs, beaten
3 tablespoons honey

Warm the liquid milk. Stir in dry milk and blend with peanut butter until smooth. Mix in eggs and honey, and pour into greased custard cups. Set the cups in a pan of hot water. (Water should come up to the same level as the custard.) Bake at 325°F for 30 minutes or until a knife inserted in the center comes out clean. Refrigerate and serve cold.

Bread Omelet

2 tablespoons bread crumbs
2 tablespoons milk
1 egg, separated
½ teaspoon butter or margarine

Mix the bread crumbs and milk. Soak for 15 minutes or overnight in a covered bowl in the refrigerator. In another bowl, beat the egg yolk well. In a third bowl, beat the egg white until stiff but not dry. Add the yolk to the bread-crumb mixture and fold in the beaten whites. Cook in a small or medium-size greased frying pan until mixture is set on the top and browned on the bottom. Remove and serve with butter, jelly, or honey. Optional additions include bacon bits and pieces of leftover meat.

Egg Posies

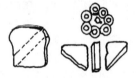

1 hard-cooked egg
1 slice bread, toasted and buttered
jelly

If you happen to have a special tool for slicing hard-cooked eggs into uniform rounds, your child can probably perform this job for you. If you don't have this gadget, use a serrated knife to slice the eggs (the short way) into ¼-inch slices. Arrange the slices at the top of a medium-size plate so they overlap and form a flower. Add a dab of jelly in the center. To make the leaves and stem, cut the slice of buttered toast into two triangles and one long strip. Arrange as shown. Voila!

Hint: If you have trouble with hard-cooked eggs coming out right, try this method: Place eggs in a deep pot. Add cold water to 1 inch higher than the tops of the eggs. Heat to boiling, then remove the pan from the burner and let the eggs set in the hot water for 15 minutes. Cool the eggs under cold running water, then refrigerate and use as needed.

Humpty Dumpty's Reprieve

Scrambled eggs are generally acceptable to the under-five crowd. Here are a few items to add a little variety to this old favorite:
- A sprinkling of wheat germ
- Crisp bacon, leftover meats, or cooked vegetables
- Cottage cheese or any grated cheese
- Drained canned corn (Heat in pan first and then add eggs.)
- Sautéed onion, celery, and/or green pepper
- Seasoned salad croutons

Green Eggs and Ham (Thank you, Dr. Seuss!)

You only need one or two drops of blue or green food coloring to turn scrambled eggs green. Or you can try the hard-cooked version: Crack the shell of a hard-cooked egg but leave it attached to the egg. Place the cracked egg in water with green food coloring for 10 minutes. When the shell is removed, you'll have a green marbled egg.

Another option is to separate egg whites from yolks. Add a few drops of green food coloring to egg whites and whisk until blended. Gently fry egg whites in a nonstick pan for 20 seconds. Then add yolks and cover until whites (now green) and yolks are firm.

Breakfast Fruit Combinations

Vitamin C is an important part of breakfast, but it need not always be served in the traditional form of orange juice. Consider the following alternatives:
- Apricots and cottage cheese
- Cantaloupe slices
- Grapes, apples, and other fruit with cheese chunks
- Mandarin oranges with sour cream or yogurt

- Orange slices cut into circles
- Sliced peaches and blueberries
- Strawberries and pineapple chunks

When serving an orange, roll it on the counter prior to cutting. It'll taste juicier. Orange juice is best when freshly squeezed, but frozen is cheaper. Make sure orange juice cans say "juice" (not "drink") and "no sugar added." If your child avoids milk and dairy products, orange juice with calcium is a good alternative.

From the Griddle

Pancakes and waffles are lots of fun for the whole family. There are prepared mixes and frozen options you can buy, which are real timesavers. If you do have the time, here are some basic recipes that could easily become traditional elements of your weekend breakfasts.

Buttermilk Beauties

1 cup flour (white, whole wheat, or a combination)
1 teaspoon baking powder
½ teaspoon baking soda
1 cup buttermilk (or use plain yogurt, plus sweet milk or water, to make 1 cup liquid)
1 tablespoon butter or margarine, melted, or vegetable oil
1 egg

Mix dry ingredients. Add milk and butter or margarine to egg, and mix. Combine the two mixtures until they're barely moistened. Bake on a hot griddle, browning both sides.

Great Groovy Griddle Cakes

1½ cups flour (white, whole wheat, or a combination)
1¾ teaspoons baking powder
2 eggs
3 tablespoons sugar or honey
3 tablespoons butter or margarine, melted, or vegetable oil
1–1¼ cups milk

Combine dry ingredients in a large bowl. Beat eggs; add sugar, butter or margarine, and milk. Add wet ingredients to dry ingredients and mix until barely moistened. Ignore the lumps. Bake on a lightly greased griddle or frying pan. When bubbles appear on upper surface of the cakes, turn and brown on other side.

Cottage-Cheese Pancakes

3 eggs
1 cup cottage cheese
2 tablespoons butter or margarine, melted
2 tablespoons flour or cornmeal

Beat eggs with a small mixer (or blender). Add cottage cheese and mix until fairly smooth. Add butter or margarine and flour. Make cakes on the "smallish" side. Bake as usual for pancakes. Great for the child who has a limited protein intake.

Personalized Pancakes

Children starting to learn letters and numbers are thrilled to have a stack of pancakes with their initials or ages on the top of each cake. Offer this on birthday mornings or to celebrate a newly learned letter or number. Here's how you do it:

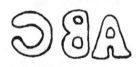

Dip a teaspoon into pancake batter and let excess drip off. With remaining batter, tip the spoon and draw the letter or number *backward* on the hot, greased pan or griddle. (You might need to practice your mirror writing on paper first!) When the underside is lightly browned, pour a spoonful of regular batter over the letter or number so the pancake completely surrounds it. Bake until bubbles appear; then turn and brown second side. The letter or number will appear darker on the finished pancake.

Or try Animal Pancakes, like this:

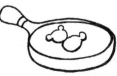

Crumpets

"Tea and crumpets" is an expression that crops up fairly regularly in English novels and films. This recipe creates one of many varieties.

3 cups flour (white, whole wheat, or a combination)
1 tablespoon baking powder
2 tablespoons sugar or honey
2 tablespoons butter or margarine
1 egg
½–1¾ cups milk

Mix flour, baking powder, and sugar. Cut in butter or margarine until mixture is like bread crumbs. Beat egg with milk. Combine wet and dry ingredients and stir just enough to moisten. (The batter should be thick, but if it doesn't spread when dropped on the griddle, add some more milk.) Drop batter by tablespoons onto hot, greased griddle. Bake as usual for pancakes.

Thin any leftover batter with a bit more milk to make larger cakes. Use instead of bread for a sandwich.

Wonderful Waffles

2 eggs, separated
4–6 tablespoons butter or margarine, melted, or vegetable oil
2 tablespoons sugar or honey
2 cups milk
2 cups flour (white, whole wheat, or a combination)
2 teaspoons baking powder

Beat egg yolks, then mix with butter or margarine and honey (if you're using it) and milk. Mix dry and liquid ingredients just enough to blend them. Beat egg whites until stiff and fold into batter. Bake according to manufacturer's instructions for your waffle iron.

Make additional waffles from your leftover batter and freeze them for later use. All you need to do is pop them in a toaster prior to eating. Or, if you're super-organized, make the whole batch ahead of time and freeze them for a series of yummy, fast breakfasts.

Variations on the Pancake or Waffle Theme

To the batter add:
• Fresh or frozen drained berries and a little extra sweetening (If possible, let batter sit ½ hour when adding fresh berries.)
• Chopped nutmeats (Again, let sit ½ hour, if possible.)
• Grated orange rind
• Finely diced ham or bacon
• Nonfat dry milk

Or:
• Replace part of the flour called for with soy flour, wheat germ, brewer's yeast, protein powder, or cornmeal for more nutritional value.
• Divide batter and add a few drops of food coloring to each batch, so you can offer a colored collection on a platter.
• For waffles, pour batter and then place a piece of uncooked bacon on batter in each section of the iron. Close iron and bake as usual.

Suggested toppings for pancakes and waffles:
• Cinnamon mixed with sugar or honey
• Peanut butter and jelly or honey
• Ice cream topped with wheat germ
• Sweetened applesauce mixed with sour cream or yogurt
• Canned or fresh fruits, such as peaches, berries, or bananas (Roll pancakes around any of the above fruits, secure with a toothpick, and serve the "logs" with syrup and butter.)
• Or the traditional maple syrup or honey and butter

French Toast

French toast is a good way to combine eggs, milk, and bread. If you're going to use homemade whole-grain bread for this purpose, be very careful as you lift the bread slices from the egg-milk mixture into the pan. Whole-grain bread is usually more fragile than white bread after being soaked.

Here are two batter recipes:

1 egg
⅓ cup milk
⅛ teaspoon vanilla

Or:

1 egg
4 teaspoons flour
⅓ cup milk

For both recipes, beat egg lightly and add next two ingredients. Dip bread into mixture. Fry in a well-greased pan over fairly high heat, browning well on both sides. Or, on a cold morning, preheat the oven to 500°F and bake the dipped bread on a greased pan, turning after the tops brown. Makes approximately 3 slices each. Serve with any of the suggested toppings for pancakes and waffles. (See page 71.)

French–Toast Waffles

1 egg, beaten
¼ cup milk
2 tablespoons butter or margarine, melted, or vegetable oil
½ teaspoon cinnamon
1–2 tablespoons sugar or honey (optional)
bread slices

Combine all ingredients, except bread, and mix well. Cut bread to fit the waffle iron. Dip bread into the batter and bake on a hot, greased iron until well browned. (It may be necessary to hold the top of the iron down for a little while, since the bread has more height than batter alone.)

French Pancakes

1 slice bread (preferably whole wheat)
1 egg
¼ teaspoon vanilla or maple extract
1 tablespoon milk

Combine ingredients in a blender. Whir until smooth.
Cook like regular pancakes.

Cereals

Cereal is one of the first foods we give our children, and
it generally continues in their diet as a breakfast staple.
Historically, cereal began as a nourishing, whole-grain
breakfast food. Processing has changed its food value,
but not the tradition. Much has been published about the
lack of nutritional value in highly processed dry cereals
on the market. Although a child does get some vitamins
and minerals, as the cereal manufacturers state, most of
the nutritional value comes from the accompanying serving of milk. Some manufacturers spray their cereals with
additional vitamins, giving you virtual vitamin pellets,
which are not a good substitute for a whole-grain or
unprocessed cereal. If you buy fortified breakfast cereals, you may be paying dearly for a few cents' worth of
vitamins. According to the Center for Science in the
Public Interest in Washington, D.C., Total, for instance, is
the same product as Wheaties, except for the sprayed-
on vitamins. Note the difference in the prices of these
products. Read your cereal labels!

Also, you'll find that many of today's popular cereals
are laden with sugar—a poor way to start off the day.
The sugar in many of the dry cereals tends to encourage
children to expect sweets along with the main part
of breakfast (as well as with other meals). In general,
avoid cereals that are sugar frosted, honey coated,
or chocolate flavored.

Some cereals that contain no sugars are Cream of Wheat (farina), Quaker Oats, Shredded Wheat, Nutri-Grain, Kretschmer Wheat Germ, and Wheatena. For more information on cereals, read Vicki Lansky's *Taming of the C.A.N.D.Y. Monster* (Book Peddlers).

Hot Cereal

You'll find many kinds of hot, cooked cereals on the market, such as Malt-O-Meal, Roman Meal, Cream of Wheat, Cream of Rice, Oatmeal (the old-fashioned variety), and others. These can be pepped up to look and taste better in any of the following ways:
- Hide one or two chocolate chips in a bowl of cereal for a bit of adventure.
- Add a heaping teaspoon of creamy peanut butter.
- Add raisins, dates, drained canned fruit, frozen fruit, or fresh fruit.
- Use any of the above to create a design on the bowl of cereal, such as a face (raisins for eyes and nose, and peach slices for mouth and ears). Draw a spiral design of jelly, or a lacy design à la Jackson Pollock, by drizzling some molasses from a spoon. Use your imagination!
- Add wheat germ, cooked soy grits, and/or nonfat dry milk.
- Serve with a large spoonful of vanilla yogurt.

Homemade Whole-Grain Easy-to-Eat Cereal

1¼ cups whole grain (brown rice, old-fashioned oats, barley, or millet)
1–1¼ cups water

Grind grain in a blender for 1–2 minutes until finely ground. Bring water to a boil in a small saucepan. Turn heat to low and add ground grain, stirring with a whisk. Cover and cook about 10 minutes, stirring often to prevent lumps and scorching.

Homemade Hot Rice Cereal

Grind several cups of raw rice (brown or white) to a fine powder in a blender. Store in a tightly covered container. To prepare:

½ cup rice powder
2 cups milk
dash of salt

In a small saucepan, bring milk and salt just to boiling point. Add rice powder, stirring constantly. Lower heat, cover pan, and simmer for 8–10 minutes. Serve with butter or margarine, honey, molasses, wheat germ, fruit, or whatever your family likes. It has a nutty taste.

Corn-off-the-Cob Hot Cereal

¼ cup yellow cornmeal
¼ cup cold water
2 teaspoons wheat germ (optional)
¾ cup boiling water
¼ cup nonfat dry milk (optional)

Mix cornmeal, cold water, and wheat germ (if you're using it). Bring ¾ cup water to a boil and add the cornmeal mixture and dry milk (if you're using it). Stirring constantly, bring to a boil and let boil about 2 minutes. Cool and serve with any of the following: butter, margarine, cottage cheese, sour cream, yogurt, jam, honey, brown sugar, maple syrup, raisins, or chopped dates.

Cold Cereal

One idea for making a nutritious and easy bowl of cereal is to crumble a whole-grain muffin in a bowl. Pour milk over it, add fruit, nuts, or sweetener, and you have an instant breakfast.

A popular natural cold cereal on the shelves is granola, which is marketed under a variety of names and variations.

Check the list of ingredients carefully, since many granolas have a high sugar and high fat content. Better yet, try making your own. It's easy, cheaper, and the proportions of ingredients can be changed to fit your family's preferences. It can also be ground in a blender and served with milk to toddlers and young children who would choke on the unground cereal. Another way to soften granola is to let it sit in a bowl of milk overnight in the refrigerator.

Granola

4 cups oatmeal, uncooked
1½ cups wheat germ (raw or toasted)
1 cup coconut, grated
¼ cup nonfat dry milk
1–2 teaspoons cinnamon
1 tablespoon brown sugar
⅓ cup vegetable oil
½ cup honey
1 tablespoon vanilla
½ cup sesame seeds (optional)
½ cup raw nuts, seeds, or raisins (optional)

Mix dry ingredients in a large bowl. Combine oil, honey, and vanilla in a saucepan and warm. Add these to the dry ingredients and stir until all particles are coated. (Hand mixing works well here.) Spread mixture in a long, low pan or rimmed baking sheet that has been greased. Bake at either 250°F for an hour or 300°F for half an hour, depending on your schedule. (Or microwave in a low glass pan for 10–15 minutes on high, stirring every 5 minutes.) Turn with a spatula from time to time. When finished toasting, add seeds, nuts, and dried fruits such as raisins. Cool and store in an airtight container.

Wheat Germ

Raw wheat germ has greater nutritional value than the toasted kind, but is less palatable. It's probably preferable to use the toasted kind as a breakfast cereal to make sure your kids will like it. Several brands are available, including some with ingredients such as honey and cinnamon. Serve any of these as regular cereal with milk (without making a big to-do about it) and see how your kids react.

If you use raw wheat germ in your cooking and want to toast your own, here's one way to do it:

4 cups raw wheat germ (always kept in refrigerator)
½ cup honey (warmed a bit)

Mix thoroughly and spread mixture on a well-greased baking sheet. Bake at 300°F for 10 minutes in bottom third of oven. Cool and store in airtight container in refrigerator.

Additional serving ideas:
- Sprinkle onto peanut-butter sandwiches.
- Mix with other sandwich fillings.
- Add to meat loaf (approximately ¼ cup).
- Toss a little in a green salad.

Rice Pudding

Usually eaten as a hearty dessert, rice pudding is a nice change of pace for breakfast that includes milk, eggs, and a grain.

2 cups cooked rice (white or brown)
2 cups milk
½ cup nonfat dry milk
¼ cup brown sugar
1 tablespoon butter or margarine, melted
2 eggs, well beaten
½ lemon rind, grated
½ teaspoon vanilla
¼ cup raisins
bread crumbs or toasted wheat germ

Mix all ingredients except bread crumbs or wheat germ. Grease a 1-quart casserole dish (or individual custard cups) and sprinkle bottom with bread crumbs or wheat germ. Pour in pudding mixture and sprinkle more crumbs on top. Bake at 350°F for 20–30 minutes or until a knife inserted in the center comes out clean. (For children, this is best prepared in advance and served cold.)

Breakfast Cookies

Although you may not want to make a regular practice of it, nutritious cookies can be a fun and interesting breakfast as well as a good snack or dessert. Many cookie recipes can be thinned with a little milk and baked in a square pan to make bars, so you have two versions of the same recipe.

Bacon-'n'-Egg Cookies

1¼ cup flour (white or whole wheat)
⅔ cup brown sugar
½ cup Grape-Nuts cereal
½ pound bacon, cooked crisp and crumbled
½ cup butter or margarine, melted
1 egg, beaten
2 tablespoons frozen orange juice concentrate, undiluted
1 tablespoon orange peel, grated

Mix flour, sugar, Grape-Nuts, and bacon. Add remaining ingredients and blend well. Drop by tablespoonfuls onto an ungreased baking sheet and bake at 350°F for 10–12 minutes or until cookies are light brown.

Banana Oatmeal Cookies

¾ cup butter or margarine
1 cup brown sugar
1 egg, beaten
1½ cups flour (white, whole wheat, or a combination)
½ teaspoon baking soda
1 teaspoon cinnamon
¼ teaspoon nutmeg

1 cup mashed banana
1¾ cups oatmeal, uncooked
optional: raisins, nuts, wheat germ, sunflower seeds, grated
   orange peel

Cream butter or margarine with sugar. Add egg and mix well. Mix flour, baking soda, cinnamon, and nutmeg and add to creamed mixture. Blend until smooth. Add mashed banana and oatmeal next. Blend. Drop by teaspoonfuls onto a greased baking sheet and bake at 400°F for 12–15 minutes.

Oatmeal Overnight Cookies

4 cups oatmeal, uncooked
2 cups brown sugar
1 cup vegetable oil
2 eggs, beaten
1 teaspoon flavoring (vanilla or almond)
¼ cup wheat germ (optional)

In the evening, combine oatmeal, brown sugar, and oil. The next morning, add eggs, flavoring, and wheat germ (if desired). Mix well. Drop by spoonfuls onto a greased baking sheet and bake at 300°F for 12–15 minutes. Watch cookies carefully. Remove from sheet while still warm or you may never get them off!

Granola Breakfast Bars

2 cups granola
2 eggs, beaten
dash of vanilla (optional)

Combine granola and eggs in a greased 8-by-8-inch pan. Bake at 350°F for 15 minutes. Cut into 8 bars. When serving, spread with jam, honey, or peanut butter.

Cereal Balls

1 cup cereal, ground (such as shredded wheat, granola,
  or wheat germ)
1 tablespoon honey
1 tablespoon peanut butter (optional)
milk (as much as needed)

After grinding cereal, add honey and peanut butter.
Blend. Add milk until mixture can be rolled into balls.
Refrigerate in a covered container.

Variations:
* Roll into logs, then roll logs in coconut or wheat germ.
* Use nonfat dry milk and brown sugar instead of
  peanut butter, liquid milk, and honey. Store in a plastic
  bag for a convenient treat while traveling. Add water
  as needed for a breakfast food or snack.

Creamy Balls

Combine chopped nuts and cream cheese. Roll into
balls and serve.

Quick Breads

If the quick breads in your repertoire of family favorites
call for white flour, try substituting whole-wheat flour. Or
use the Cornell Triple-Rich Formula (page 84) with the
flour you're using. When substituting whole-grain flour
for white, use more baking powder since whole grains
require a bit more help in rising.

Breakfast Banana-Nut Bread

¼ cup butter or margarine
½ cup brown sugar
1 egg, beaten
1 cup bran cereal or oatmeal, uncooked
4–5 ripe bananas (about 1½ cups), mashed
1 teaspoon vanilla

1½ cups flour (white, whole wheat, or a combination)
2 teaspoons baking powder
½ teaspoon baking soda
½ cup nuts, chopped

Cream butter or margarine and sugar until light. Add egg and mix well. Stir in cereal, bananas, and vanilla. Combine the remaining ingredients in a bowl and add to the first mixture, stirring just enough to moisten the flour. Grease and flour a loaf pan. Pour in batter. Bake at 350°F for 1 hour or until bread tests done.

Hint: Wondering what to do with that leftover ripe banana? Mash it, add a bit of lemon juice or Fruit-Fresh, and freeze it until it's time to make banana bread. If chopped nuts aren't appropriate for your child, whirl them in a blender before adding to batter.

Peanut–Butter Bread

2 cups flour (white, whole wheat, or a combination)
4 teaspoons baking powder
¼ cup sugar or honey
⅔ cup peanut butter
1¼ cups milk

Lightly mix dry ingredients in a large bowl. If using honey, cream it with peanut butter in a separate bowl. Heat the milk until lukewarm, then add peanut butter and blend well. Add the wet and dry ingredients and beat thoroughly. Pour into a greased loaf pan and bake at 350°F for 45–50 minutes. When the bread is cold, make thin slices and spread with honey or jam. (Bread slices best if baked a day in advance and refrigerated after cooking.)

Ready Bran Muffins

2 cups boiling water
6 cups 100 percent bran cereal
1 cup butter or margarine
2 cups sugar or 1⅔ cups honey

4 eggs, beaten
1 quart buttermilk
5 cups flour (white, whole wheat, or a combination)
5 teaspoons baking soda
optional: blueberries, raisins, coconut, peanuts, chopped fresh
    apples, chopped dates, nuts

Preheat oven to 375°F. Pour boiling water over 2 cups of cereal and set aside. Cream butter or margarine with sugar or honey and add eggs, buttermilk, and moistened bran cereal. Mix. Fold in the remaining dry ingredients. Fill greased muffin tins ¾-full and bake 20–25 minutes. Or fill a loaf pan ½-full and bake at 350°F until done. Batter can be stored in quart jars in the refrigerator for up to six weeks.

Hint: The proportions called for in this recipe make several quarts of batter. If that's too much, cut the recipe in half, give some to a neighbor, or store some in the freezer.

Whole-Wheat Muffins

1 cup whole-wheat flour
¾ cup white flour
¼ cup sugar or honey
4 teaspoons baking powder
1 egg
1 cup milk
¼ cup vegetable oil

Mix dry ingredients. In a separate bowl, beat egg slightly and stir in milk and oil. Add wet ingredients to dry ingredients and stir until barely moistened. Batter will be lumpy. Fill greased muffin tins ⅔-full and bake at 400°F for 20–25 minutes. Remove muffins from tins immediately after baking.

Orange Muffins

1 slice bread (preferably whole grain)
1 egg

⅓ cup nonfat dry milk
½ teaspoon baking soda
1 orange, peeled and cut up
1 tablespoon water
4 teaspoons honey or sugar

Put the bread in a bowl and pull apart with a fork. Mix remaining ingredients and combine with bread. Spoon into greased muffin cups until ⅔-full. Bake at 350°F for 30 minutes.

Quickie Turnovers

1 8-ounce can refrigerated crescent rolls

Filling:
   ½ cup honey
   1 tablespoon sunflower seeds
   1 tablespoon raisins
   ¼ cup blueberries

Combine all filling ingredients. Unroll crescent rolls and place a spoonful of filling mixture in the middle of each triangle of dough. Moisten the edges of the dough with a bit of water or milk. Following the diagram above, fold point A over to point C. Press edges firmly together. Place on a greased baking sheet and bake at 375°F for 10–12 minutes.

Filling variations:
   peanut butter
   jelly
   nonfat dry milk
   raisins

Or:
   honey
   granola
   apple slices
   cinnamon and nuts
   bread

Bread

The art of baking bread is coming back into its own in the United States. If you've never tried it, why not start now? The aroma of yeast bread baking is a delight, one to which you and your family could take a real liking. You'll need to carve out time slots that include 5–10 minutes of concentrated work spread over several hours.

Batter breads are somewhat simpler than breads that must be kneaded, so try a batter recipe if you're a new bread baker. If baking bread just isn't your thing, consider using frozen bread dough from your grocer's freezer section. You merely let it thaw and rise, then bake. Most frozen doughs don't contain the extra ingredients that make bread shelf-stable, but the bread tastes and smells so good that it disappears very quickly. The major disadvantage of this type of bread is that it's difficult to slice into thin pieces.

You've probably noticed throughout this book that when flour is called for, the recipe generally gives you a choice of white, whole wheat, or a combination of the two. Here's what the authors of *The Joy of Cooking* have to say about bleached, enriched white flour: "After the removal of the outer coats and germ, our flours may be enriched, but the term is misleading. Enriched flours contain only four of the many ingredients known to have been removed from it in the milling." You can give additional nutritional value to white flour for cakes, cookies, muffins, and breads by using the simple method below.

Cornell Triple-Rich Formula

1 tablespoon soy flour
1 tablespoon nonfat dry milk
1 teaspoon raw wheat germ

Place these ingredients in the bottom of your measuring cup before adding flour. Then add flour to make one cup. Do this for each cup of flour you use. Eventually you may want to add a little more of each enriching ingredient. Whole-grain flours also benefit from this formula.

Bread-Making Procedures

If you're wondering how to tell if bread dough or batter has doubled in bulk, there's an easy way to find out. Press lightly with one or two fingers near the edge of the dough. If a small indentation remains, it has doubled. If the dough springs back, it hasn't.

When bread is browning too quickly (turning a light brown after only 10–15 minutes), cover the top lightly with a piece of aluminum foil.

If you've never kneaded, don't let that stop you. You'll improve with practice, so start experimenting now. Kneading is a process of folding the dough and pressing it down with the heel of your hand, over and over again, until the dough is smooth and elastic, not sticky. You may need to sprinkle flour on the dough and your working surface when you begin until the dough loses some of its stickiness.

If you need a warm place to let your bread rise without busy little fingers reaching for it, place a baking pan filled with about an inch of hot water on the bottom shelf of your oven. Put the bowl or pans of rising dough on the middle shelf. You may have to replace the water every half hour or so. Don't forget to remove the pan of water when you bake your bread! Another option is to heat your oven to 200°F for 60 seconds, turn it off, then put in the bread for rising.

Basic Whole-Wheat Bread

2 packages yeast
1 cup warm water (105°F–115°F)
1 tablespoon honey
2 cups milk
¼ cup butter, margarine, or vegetable oil
⅓ cup honey
1½ tablespoons salt
5 cups whole-wheat flour
¼ cup wheat germ (optional)
3 cups white flour

Dissolve yeast in warm water. Stir in 1 tablespoon honey. Set aside for 10 minutes. In a saucepan, combine milk, butter (or margarine or oil), honey, and salt. Heat to luke-warm—do not scald. Pour warm milk mixture and dissolved yeast into a large mixing bowl. Add the whole-wheat flour, one cup at a time, beating well after each addition. Be sure to use all the whole-wheat flour. Add wheat germ, if desired.

Add enough white flour to make a soft, yet manageable, dough. Turn out on a lightly floured board and knead until smooth and elastic (approximately 8–10 minutes). Place dough in a greased bowl, turning it to grease the top. Cover and let rise in a warm, draft-free place until dough has doubled in bulk. Punch down, divide in half, and knead each half for about 30 seconds. Shape into three loaves and place in greased loaf pans. Cover and let rise again until doubled in bulk, about 45 minutes. Preheat oven to 400°F and bake 40 minutes or until done.

Cinnamon Swirl Bread

Follow the above dough recipe, but before shaping the dough, roll into three rectangles, about 6-by-16-inches each. Mix 4 tablespoons brown sugar and 4 tablespoons cinnamon. Sprinkle ¼ cup of this mixture over each rectangle. Beginning with the narrow side, roll up tightly into a loaf. Seal ends and bottom by pinching dough together to make a seam. Place in the loaf pans and proceed as in the above recipe.

Refrigerator 100 Percent Whole-Wheat Bread

5 cups milk or water
2 packages dry yeast, dissolved in 1 cup warm water (105°F –115°F)
½ cup butter or margarine, melted, or vegetable oil
¼ cup molasses
¼ cup honey
2 tablespoons salt
11–12 cups whole-wheat flour (or a combination of 9–10 cups whole-wheat and 1–2 cups soy flour)

This recipe is especially good if you work outside the home or are too busy during the day with the kids to make bread. Mix the dough in the evening, set it in the refrigerator, let it rise, and bake the next evening. If the dough is to be refrigerated for only three hours, use luke-warm liquid. If it's to be left longer, use cool liquid so dough will not rise too much. Dough may still require punching down a few times while it's in the refrigerator.

In a 6-quart pan or bowl, mix the liquid, dissolved yeast, butter or margarine, molasses, honey, and salt. Add flour gradually, mixing well after each addition. (If using soy flour, add after at least 4 cups of whole-wheat flour have been added.) This dough will be moister than ordinary bread dough. Let dough rest in the bowl for 1–15 minutes.

Turn dough out on a floured board and knead for about 10 minutes, adding as little extra flour as possible. Replace in the bowl, cover with foil or a dampened cloth, and refrigerate immediately for 3–24 hours. Remove from the refrigerator, punch down, and let stand 30–60 minutes at room temperature.

Divide into four equal portions, shape into loaves, and place in four well-greased loaf pans. (See hint below.) Lightly grease the tops of the loaves. Let rise in a warm, draft-free place until almost doubled in bulk. Preheat oven to 425°F, place pans in oven, reduce heat to 325°F, and bake for 1 hour or until done.

Note: This dough makes excellent hamburger buns. Use ¼–⅓ cup dough for each bun. Bake at 325°F for 25–30 minutes or until done.

Hint: If your oven won't hold four pans at one time or you don't own four pans, remove only enough dough from the refrigerator as you can bake at one time. But make sure to take the rest out and use it within twenty-four hours.

Swiss–Cheese Bread

This bread tastes very nearly like a grilled Swiss-cheese sandwich when toasted. And its braided, glazed top makes it very pretty!

1½ cups milk
2 tablespoons sugar or honey
1 tablespoon salt
2 tablespoons butter, margarine, or vegetable oil
2 cups grated Swiss cheese (8 ounces)
2 packages dry yeast
½ cup warm water (105°F–115°F)
5 cups white flour (approximately)

Preheat oven to 350°F. Scald milk and combine with sugar or honey, salt, butter or margarine, and cheese in a large bowl. (Cheese will probably melt into a lump, but don't worry.) Let cool until lukewarm. Dissolve yeast in the warm water and add to the cooled milk mixture. Stir well. Gradually add flour, stirring well after each addition until a fairly stiff dough is formed.

Knead dough about 5–8 minutes. Place in a greased bowl, turning to grease top. Let it rise in a warm, draft-free place until doubled in bulk. Punch down and divide the dough into two equal portions. Roll each piece out into an 11-by-15-inch rectangle. Cut each rectangle into three equal strips (the long way), leaving the strips joined at one end. Braid the strips loosely. Pinch the three ends together. Place each braided loaf in a well-greased pan. Cover and let rise until doubled. Bake 40–45 minutes.

Variation: Just before popping loaves in the oven, beat an egg with 1 tablespoon cool water and brush on tops of loaves. Sprinkle on poppy or sesame seeds.

Triple-Rich-Batter White Bread

A good choice for a new baker.

1 cup milk
3 tablespoons sugar or honey
1 tablespoon salt
2 tablespoons butter or margarine, melted, or vegetable oil
2 packages dry yeast

1 cup warm water (105°F–115°F)
4¼ cups white flour, unsifted
Cornell Triple-Rich Formula (page 84)

Scald milk. Stir in sugar or honey, salt, and butter or margarine. Set aside to cool until lukewarm (105°F–115°F). Add yeast to warm water in a large bowl and stir until dissolved. Pour warm milk mixture into the yeast. Stir in the flour, one cup at a time, placing the Cornell Triple-Rich Formula in the bottom of the measuring cup first. Beat with a long-handled spoon for about 2 minutes, or longer if using whole-wheat flour.

Cover with a cloth and let rise in a warm, draft-free place until more than doubled in bulk (about 40 minutes). Stir batter down and beat vigorously for about 30 seconds. Grease two loaf pans (9-by-5-by-3-inch). Divide batter evenly between them. Batter does not need to rise again. Preheat oven to 375°F and bake for about 50 minutes.

Variations:
- Try using part or all whole-wheat flour. Beat a minute or two longer than for white flour.
- Add one or more beaten eggs for a different texture.

Raisin-'n'-Egg-Batter Bread

This bread has a rich, cakelike quality.

1 cup milk
½ cup sugar or honey
1 teaspoon salt
¼ cup butter or margarine or vegetable oil
2 packages dry yeast
½ cup warm water (105°F–115°F)
1 egg, beaten
4½ cups white flour
1 cup raisins
Cornell Triple-Rich Formula (page 84), optional

Preheat oven to 350°F. Scald milk. Stir in sugar or honey, salt, and butter or margarine. Let cool to lukewarm (105°F–115°F). Add yeast to warm water in a large bowl and stir until dissolved. Pour the warm milk mixture into the yeast. Add the egg, then mix in 3 cups of flour, beating well after each addition. After the third cup, beat until smooth. Stir in remaining flour to make a stiff batter.

Cover with a cloth and let rise in a warm, draft-free place until doubled in bulk (about 1 hour). Stir batter down and beat in raisins, distributing them as evenly as possible. Grease 2 1-quart casserole dishes or 2 loaf pans, and divide the batter evenly between them. Batter does not need to rise again. Bake for 40–45 minutes or until done.

English Muffins

This is a good summer option because you don't have to turn on the oven.

> 1 cup milk, scalded
> 2 tablespoons sugar or honey
> ¼ cup butter or margarine or vegetable oil
> 1 tablespoon salt
> 1 package dry yeast
> 1 cup warm water (105°F–115°F)
> 5–6 cups flour (white, whole wheat, or a combination)
> cornmeal

Place hot milk in a large bowl and add sugar or honey, butter or margarine, and salt. Let cool to lukewarm. Dissolve yeast in the warm water and add to the cooled milk. Add 3 cups of flour and beat until smooth. Gradually add more flour, beating well after each addition until a soft dough is formed.

Turn out on a lightly floured board and knead until smooth and elastic (8–10 minutes), adding more flour as necessary. Place in a greased bowl, turning to grease the top. Cover and let rise in a warm, draft-free place until doubled in bulk (about 1 hour). Punch down and divide in half.

On a lightly floured board, roll the first half out to about ½-inch thickness and cut as many circles of dough as you can with a muffin cutter. (See hint below.) Gently remove to a baking sheet that has been heavily sprinkled with cornmeal. Sprinkle tops with cornmeal, too. Push scraps together, roll out, and cut again. Continue until you use all the dough. Cover the muffins with a cloth and let rise until doubled.

To bake, heat a griddle or electric frying pan to moderately hot (about 300°F) and grease lightly. Using a large spatula, move as many muffins as will fit (without touching) to the griddle. Bake until bottoms are browned (10–15 minutes). Then turn and bake other sides. To cut, insert tines of fork all the way around and pull apart with your fingers.

Hint: A 7-ounce tuna-type can with both ends removed is a perfect cutter for the muffins. But for fun, try cutting them with large, not-too-detailed cookie cutters. (Some won't keep their shape; some will.)

Bagels

1½ cups warm water (105°F–115°F)
1 package dry yeast
1 tablespoon salt
3 tablespoons sugar or honey
4–6 cups flour (white, whole wheat, or a combination)
1 egg
poppy or sesame seeds (optional)

Preheat oven to 375°F. In a large bowl, mix warm water with yeast. Add salt and sugar (or honey). Cover bowl and let stand 5 minutes. Gradually add flour until a soft-to-medium (but not stiff) dough is obtained. Knead on a lightly floured board (5–10 minutes) until shiny and smooth. Add a little more flour as necessary for kneading. Place in a greased bowl, turning to grease the top.

Cover and let rise in a warm, draft-free place until doubled (about 30 minutes). Punch down and knead lightly.

To shape into bagels, roll approximately ¼ cup dough into a strand about 7 inches long and pinch the ends firmly together. Place bagels fairly close together on a floured board or baking sheet. Cover and let rise again (about 30 minutes) in a warm place.

In the meantime, bring about 5 inches of water to boil in a fairly large, open kettle. Turn heat down so water is simmering. When bagels have risen, gently lift one at a time and drop into the simmering water. Turn them immediately and simmer for about 2 minutes until puffy but not disintegrating. Several bagels may be put in the water at one time, but do not crowd the pan. Remove the bagels to a towel-covered area to drain and cool while you're boiling the next batch. Place cooled bagels on a greased baking sheet. They can be close together.

Beat the egg briefly with 1 tablespoon of cool water and brush mixture over the tops of the bagels. Sprinkle with poppy or sesame seeds, if desired. Bake for 30–40 minutes. This procedure may look complicated at first, but once you get the knack, you can turn out a batch in 3–3½ hours, from start to finish. Makes 12–15 bagels.

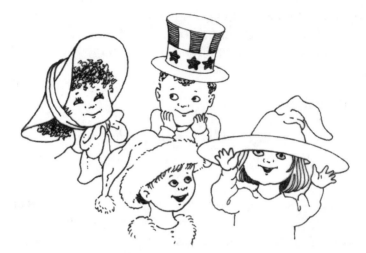

Chapter Six
Seasonal Recipes

Here are some seasonal ideas that are often more fun than nutritious, but worth trying on occasion. Many of these recipes yield sugary treats that should be served in moderation.

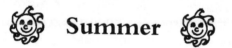

Summer

Summer means little hands constantly opening the refrigerator in search of things to quench thirst and hunger.

Yogurt Popsicles

1 carton vanilla yogurt
1 6-ounce can concentrated fruit juice, unsweetened
  (Orange seems to be a favorite.)
dash of vanilla and/or honey (optional)

Mix well and freeze in molds. (Three-ounce paper cups work well.) For handles, insert wooden sticks or spoons when mixture is partially frozen.

Variation: Make single servings by mixing some plain yogurt with puréed canned or ripe fruit (or a spoonful of jam or jelly) in a small paper cup. Add a bit of vanilla for extra sweetness, if needed.

Fudgesicles

1 4-ounce package regular chocolate pudding mix
3½ cups skim milk
1 egg (optional)

Prepare pudding according to instructions on box. Sweeten to taste. (An egg may be added for extra nutritional value.) Freeze in molds or paper cups. When partially frozen, insert Popsicle sticks for handles.

Quickie Pops

juice (apple, pineapple, orange, or grape)
1 teaspoon vanilla ice cream, melted

Add juice and ice cream to a mold or paper cup. Mix well and freeze. Add handle when partially frozen. This has the advantage of allowing you to make just one or two rather than a whole batch. It's also a good way to get kids to down some juice, or to use up juice leftover from breakfast.

Variation: Mash or blend pitted watermelon cubes, pour into a mold, and freeze to make a Popsicle.

Hint: In ice cube trays, freeze juices and syrups leftover from canned fruits. Use these to "perk up" lemonade or fruit punch. Or insert sticks into cubes before freezing and use as Popsicles.

Hint: Before serving, poke the stick of any frozen pop through a flat basket-shaped coffee filter to catch inevitable drips.

Banana Pops

Peel 3 bananas and cut them in half. Push a Popsicle stick up the center of each half and freeze. Serve this way or dip in honey and roll in toasted wheat germ, nuts, or granola.

If you have the time and inclination, melt 6 ounces of chocolate chips (or 12 ounces for 6 bananas) and add a few tablespoons of water. Dip the frozen bananas in the chocolate and coat to cover. Twirl to remove excess. After the chocolate sets, wrap in foil and store in the freezer.

Hint: To use up leftover chocolate, add raisins, nuts, coconut, wheat germ, or whatever you have. Drop by teaspoonfuls on a sheet, and cool in the refrigerator for some wholesome candy.

Do-It-Yourself Ice-Cream Sandwiches

Spread softened ice cream so it completely covers one side of a cookie or graham cracker. Gently press another cookie or cracker on top. Wrap individually or stack together in foil or plastic wrap, and freeze.

Ice-cream and frozen yogurt cones are still an all-time favorite. These dairy treats at least provide needed calcium for growing kids. Choose flat-bottom cones whenever possible. If using pointed cones, try this: Punch a hole in a small foil plate or cupcake paper, and place around the cone to catch the inevitable drippings.

Fruit Ices

Base Syrup:

2 cups water
2 cups sugar

Cook on a low boil for 10 minutes or until the base is almost at the jelly stage on a candy thermometer. Cool. Use as a base for orange ice, grape ice, or lemon ice. (See page 96.)

Orange Ice

2 cups fresh orange juice
¼ cup lemon juice (or juice from 1 lemon)

Grape Ice

1½ cups grape juice
⅔ cup orange juice
3 tablespoons lemon juice

Lemon Ice

¾ cup lemon juice
1 tablespoon lemon peel, grated
2 cups water

Pour into trays or a small mixing bowl and freeze. Watch for "mushy" stage (1 hour), then stir semi-frozen mixture in the tray and refreeze. Good alone or served by the scoop in a fruit drink.

Summer Drinks

All drinks seem to disappear from the refrigerator extra fast at this time of year. The best warm-weather drinks are easy to tote and serve. Small juice cans and disposable boxes of drinks work well. But beverages, like everything else, should be purchased with an eye toward nutrition. Yes, the real juice drinks cost more, but colored and flavored sugar water is still only sugar water!

Natural fruit-flavored sodas in cans and bottles are popular these days. Though thirst quenching, these have little nutritional value. Many include only 10 percent fruit juice. For the average active child, an occasional sugared soda may be preferable. If you do buy sodas, avoid ones with caffeine, since children tend to be stimulated enough already.

Keeping a good supply of drinks on hand is no easy task. Here are a few extra ideas:

Apple Juice: Try the frozen or shelf-stable concentrate. It's delicious, sugarless, and economical since it can always be stretched a bit. It can also be reconstituted with carbonated water for a change of pace.

Flavored Milk: When jam or jelly jars are almost empty, pour in cold milk. Shake and serve as a fruit-flavored drink.

Grape Juice: You can double any amount of grape juice from a bottle by adding an equal amount of water and, for each 2 cups of water added, ½ cup sugar and 1–2 fresh lemons. This takes away the "heaviness" from pure grape juice and gives you more for your money.

Fruit Drink: To a glass of lemonade or light carbonated drink, add fresh fruit (pineapple, grapes, strawberries, or other favorites) and serve with a fork or toothpick, plus a straw.

Water: Keeping cold water in the refrigerator is an excellent way to encourage consumption of this inexpensive, sugar-free beverage.

Special Touches: Increase the fun of drinks by adding interesting ice cubes. Freeze various fruit juices in ice cube trays in order to add colors and flavors to those you serve frequently, such as orange juice. Or, make ice cubes more interesting by adding a raspberry, strawberry, or blueberry to each ice cube section before adding water and freezing.

Topping a drink with whipped cream is always exciting. Add to the interest by sprinkling a few colored sprinkles on the whipped-cream topping.

Lemonade

3 lemons, sliced
1 cup sugar
ice cubes
water

Put lemons and sugar in a 2-quart pitcher or bowl. With a large spoon, pound the lemons to release their juice. Stir. Add a batch of ice cubes and let sit awhile, then add water to fill. Mix and serve.

Or try:

1 cup reconstituted lemon juice
1½ cups sugar
2 quarts water

Mix and serve.

Summer Picnics

Summer means picnics, whether you camp out or simply cook out. A backyard or park is as exciting to a child as a national park campsite may be to you. And don't forget you can use your front stoop for a picnic lunch.

You can simplify any picnic by putting your meal on a skewer. Try cubes of cheese and pieces of chicken (or any cooked meat) along with pineapple chunks, cherry tomatoes, and pickles on a stick—and then bag it! Your meal can be eaten right off the stick or slid into a hot dog bun. The same will work for dessert, whether it's cookies and marshmallows for toasting or just a selection of fruits.

Finger Jell-O (page 56) is terrific picnic fare, assuming you're not going to the desert. It doesn't melt easily. And don't overlook the magic of a marshmallow roast. Children under three years old will probably eat them uncooked off the stick and still consider it a nifty event. If it's a backyard cookout, let your child invite some friends over for a social event of their own.

Take Care

Do not let children run while eating from sticks. Also, beware of sticks with sharp points and those from unfamiliar (and possibly poisonous) trees or shrubs, such as oleander!

S'Mores

large marshmallows
Hershey bars
graham crackers

The traditional recipe! Place a toasted, softened marshmallow and 4 squares of a Hershey bar between 2 graham crackers, and you've done it!

Watermelon Carving

Don't limit your carving creativity to pumpkins. Make memorable summer shapes from this mouthwatering favorite. In addition to the common "basket" style, try faces, bunnies, racing cars, or whatever else you can think of.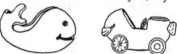

July 4th: Independence Day

This is our only major summer holiday, so add a little red-white-and-blue to your table:

• Make or buy cupcakes with white frosting, and top with several small red and/or blue birthday candles. These will simulate firecrackers when lit. (Optional: Add colored sprinkles.)
• Use your star cookie cutter to cut out pie dough to create a top star "crust" for a cherry pie.
• Make Finger Jell-O stars using red and blue Jell-O.
• Use strawberries, blueberries, mini-marshmallows, and Cool Whip (as well as mini flag toothpicks) to create patriotic dishes and toppings.
• Let your kids ride their bikes and trikes over plastic bubble wrap for safe, fireless "firecrackers."

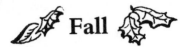 **Fall**

Apple Cider

In a saucepan: Heat apple cider, but do not boil. Add a stick of cinnamon and a few cloves.

In a coffee percolator: Put whole spices, such as stick cinnamon and cloves, in the percolator basket. Pour apple juice in the bottom container. Perk a few minutes until cider is spiced to your taste.

In a drip coffee maker: Pour cider into reservoir. Put cinnamon and/or cloves in the coffee filter basket and let it "brew."

Hot-Chocolate Mix

1 25-ounce box nonfat dry milk
1 6-ounce jar Coffee-mate
1 pound instant cocoa
1 cup sugar

Mix well. Store in a covered container. To make hot chocolate, add 3–4 tablespoons of mix to 1 cup boiling water. Stir.

Doughnuts

Use 1 package refrigerated biscuit dough. Punch a hole in the middle of each biscuit. (A bottle cap or a small, empty, circular pill container will work.) Fry in 1 inch of hot vegetable oil for about 1 minute or until lightly browned on both sides. Fry the "holes" too. When cool, shake in a bag of cinnamon mixed with sugar, brown sugar, or powdered sugar.

Popcorn

Children love any and all forms of popcorn (*although popcorn is not recommended for children under four years of age*). It's as much fun to make and watch as it is to eat. Instead of salt, sprinkle on cheese flavoring or a little butter.

TLC Peanut Butter

If you've never made your own peanut butter, now's the time to try a batch. It's a good rainy day (or any day) activity. The challenge is to shell more than you eat!

1 pound (or less) peanuts-in-the-shell
1–2 tablespoons vegetable oil
salt (optional)

Shell and then chop peanuts in a blender until fine, one cup at a time. (Or buy peanuts already shelled and toss them in a blender.) Add vegetable oil. Add salt only if peanuts are unsalted. Makes about 1 cup of delicious peanut butter that should be stored in the refrigerator. You may also want to experiment with other kinds of nuts such as almonds, cashews, or walnuts.

Spellin' Cookies

1 package gingerbread mix
⅓ cup water

With school in progress, help with the homework by making three-letter-word cookies. Combine gingerbread mix with water. Roll out on a floured surface and cut into 3-inch-round cookies. Place them on a greased baking sheet. With a knife cut the circle in thirds and push the pieces slightly apart. Bake. When cool, make three-letter words with frosting (a single letter on each piece).

Cuttin' Cookies

3 eggs, beaten
½ cup corn oil
1 cup sugar

1 teaspoon vanilla or almond flavoring
3 cups flour
1 teaspoon baking powder

Combine all ingredients. Work on a well-floured surface. Roll out and cut into shapes with cookie cutter or knife. (You may wish to chill the dough before rolling out.) Bake at 350°F for 8–10 minutes.

Variation:
½ cup butter or margarine
1 cup sugar
1 egg
1 tablespoon milk
1 teaspoon vanilla
2 cups flour
1 teaspoon baking powder
1 teaspoon nutmeg

Roll out on a floured surface. Cut into shapes. Bake on a greased baking sheet at 375°F for 6–8 minutes.

Hints:
- Consider using play-dough-shape makers for extra fun and games. Or cut around your child's hand.
- Freeze extra cookie dough in clean frozen juice cans that are open at both ends, and wrap or bag before placing in the freezer. When ready to use, push out, slice, and bake.

Easy Applesauce

several apples
¼ cup water or apple juice
cinnamon
sweetener
lemon or Fruit-Fresh

Take advantage of the fall harvest by making fresh applesauce. Peel, core, and slice several apples. In a blender pour ¼ cup water or apple juice and add apples one at a time. Blend until smooth. Pour into a saucepan and cook on low heat for 5–10 minutes. Add cinnamon and sweetener (honey or light corn syrup, for example) to taste. A dash of lemon or Fruit-Fresh will retard its "darkening" action.

Edible Decorating Glue

Spread baked cookies with a thin coating of honey. Then dip in shredded coconut, toasted wheat germ, or candy décors.

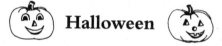 **Halloween**

Halloween is second only to Christmas in holiday excitement for your child. Full understanding of Halloween—costumes *and* candy, and not necessarily in that order—comes at a surprisingly early age.

Even if you're not planning to make a variety of Halloween food items, don't let that stop you from having fun renaming whatever you do prepare. Choose from this list for starters:

Bat Bars
Devil's Delight
Creepy Cookies
Vampire Vitals
Monster Meat (or Munchies)
Goblin Supreme
Witches Stew (or Brew)
Ghost Gourmet

You can rename peanuts-in-the-shells "Bats' Knuckles," or you can call pretzels and bread sticks "Witches Broomsticks."

To spice up any meal or snack, use your cookie cutter to make a pumpkin face in a piece of cheese or to cut a sandwich into a Halloween shape. Turn Peanut-Butter Balls (page 58) into spiders by inserting 6 2-inch pieces of string licorice. Add a minidrop of red and yellow food coloring to a glass of milk to turn it into "Pumpkin Punch."

Put a gummy worm into a small hole you cut out of an apple for a fun, "nauseating" snack.

Enjoy carving pumpkins while you can, because by the time your children are in elementary school, they'll probably take over the responsibility—and the fun. Never carve a pumpkin more than two days before Halloween, or it will shrivel up and "die." An ice-cream scoop is a good tool for extracting fiber and seeds. Enhance your jack-o'-lantern by inserting eggshell halves with eyeballs painted on them into rounded eyeholes in the pumpkin.

Use permanent markers to decorate your pumpkins in the weeks before carving, then carve and use them for cooking on or after Halloween. Use a cleaned-out pumpkin for cooking or as a serving bowl. Cookie cutters are good for tracing designs on your pumpkin. You don't have to cut off the top of the pumpkin for a lid; cut a round opening from the bottom instead. To light the pumpkin, simply lower it over a lit candle or a small flashlight.

Roll out Peanut-Butter Balls (page 58) into small snake shapes and call them "Crawlers." Instead of bobbing for apples in water, try bobbing for doughnuts hanging from strings from the top of a doorway. Remember, the trick (and fun) is NOT using hands!

Cooked Pumpkin

Use this method to cook pumpkin for a vegetable dish or pumpkin cake. Wash a pumpkin and cut it into large pieces. Remove the seeds and strings or fibers. Put pumpkin pieces, shell side up, in a baking pan at 325°F oven for 1 hour or more until pumpkin is very tender. (Microwaves can do small amounts in less time.) Scrape pulp from the shells and put it through a food mill or ricer. If the pulp isn't thick enough to stand in peaks, simmer it in a saucepan for 5–10 minutes, stirring constantly. Freeze in family-size servings.

Toasted Pumpkin Seeds

Don't throw away those wet, string-laden pumpkin seeds. They're a delicious treat! Wash the seeds and remove the strings to the best of your ability. Soak the seeds overnight in salted water (1½ teaspoons salt per ⅔ cup water). Coat the seeds lightly with vegetable oil and spread them on a low baking pan in the oven at 300°F for approximately 20 minutes or until golden. Eat with or without removing the shells. Of course, you can squirrel away a few untoasted seeds and plant them in your garden when spring comes around.

Pumpkin Fries

Cut a small, fresh pumpkin in half. Peel. Cut into matchstick slices and toss with 2–3 tablespoons of peanut oil. Bake on a baking sheet in a hot oven until brown and tender. Stir often. Sprinkle with cinnamon to taste.

Pumpkin Candy

See Fruit Roll recipe on pages 61–62. Use canned pumpkin in place of other fruits to tailor this recipe for Halloween.

Pumpkin Cup

Cut a "cap" from an orange, preferably the navel variety. Remove the inside pulp and fill with fruit or other treats. Put a toothpick, which can be used as the eating utensil, on the top of the "cap." Also, scratch a face on the orange and trace the face with a ballpoint pen so the features stand out, or use a permanent felt-tip marker.

Pumpkin Muffins

1½ cups flour
½ cup sugar
2 teaspoons baking powder
1 teaspoon cinnamon
½ teaspoon ginger
¼ teaspoon cloves
½ cup raisins

1 egg, slightly beaten
½ cup milk
½ cup solid pack pumpkin, canned
¼ cup butter or margarine, melted
2½ teaspoons sugar, mixed with ½ teaspoon cinnamon

Sift the first six ingredients into a mixing bowl. Stir in raisins. Combine egg, milk, pumpkin, and melted butter or margarine. Add wet ingredients to sifted mixture, mixing only until combined. Fill greased muffin pans ⅔-full; sprinkle with cinnamon-sugar mixture. Bake in 400°F oven for 20–25 minutes. Makes a dozen muffins.

Hint: Canned pumpkin labels often include additional recipes and cookbook offers.

Dessert Pumpkins

- To make orange frosting for cakes, cupcakes, or cookies, add equal drops of red and yellow food coloring to white frosting.
- To make black frosting, mix the following ingredients and add to white frosting:
  1½ teaspoons green food coloring
  1½ teaspoons red food coloring
  5 drops blue food coloring
- Candy corn can be used for the eyes, nose, and mouth of a "face."

Pumpkin Dessert Cake

See recipe on page 109.

Fanged Favorites

- Cut oranges into quarters and use permanent markers to draw spiked teeth on the rind, or carve them with a knife. Let your little ones sink their teeth into the meat of the orange and show off their newfound "fangs."

- Make a terrific "monster mouth" snack by spreading peanut butter on two thin wedges of red-skinned apples. Place a few mini-marshmallows between the wedges to look like teeth.
- Turn any pizza into a toothy monster face. Mushrooms, green-pepper slices, cut-up sausage, even candy corn can transform any cooked pizza into a creepy creature.

Ghostly Treats

- To one dollop of whipped-cream topping, add a smaller dollop and insert two chocolate chips for eyes. Use to top off cereals, custards, pancakes, or a fruit plate.
- Push a toothpick through two large marshmallows. Use chocolate chips, raisins, or dark tube icing for eyes.
- White frosting on any ghost-shaped cookie (plus chocolate chips for eyes) is all you need.
- Cut a banana in half and push a Popsicle stick into the cut end of each half. Dip banana in white chocolate or bark that has been melted in the microwave. Cool on wax paper or place in freezer after pressing in chocolate chips or raisins for eyes.
- Shape peanut-butter balls into ghostly shapes. Roll in flaked coconut or use a can of vanilla frosting to coat them white. (*Hint:* If you microwave frosting in a dish for 10–20 seconds, it will be runnier and easier to apply. Or thin with a bit of milk or a spoonful of white vinegar.)
- Use a ghost-shaped cookie cutter to create Ghost Toast. Make eyes by using a toothpick as a hole punch.
- Heavy mashed potatoes can also be shaped into mealtime ghosts.

Hand Horrors

- Fill a disposable, clear plastic glove (not the kind with the interior powder coating) with water, tie, and freeze. Dip the frozen glove in warm water and peel off the plastic. Float it in a party punch for a chilling effect.
- Make a fun treat by placing a piece of candy corn in the bottom of each finger of a clear plastic glove (to

107

look like fingernails). Fill the rest of the glove with popcorn or similar treats. Tie the wrist closed with a ribbon.
• Spray the inside of a plastic glove with nonstick cooking spray. Fill the glove with green Finger Jell-O (page 56). Tie glove and refrigerate. Cut away glove with scissors.

Thanksgiving

This warm, family holiday centers on a large turkey dinner, which most children thoroughly enjoy. It's traditional to stuff a turkey, as well as stuffing ourselves.

Apple Turkeys

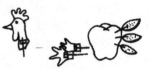

Use an apple as the "body." Cut "tail feathers" from orange peels and attach with toothpicks to the apple. Cut the "head" and "feet" from heavy paper and tape to toothpick "neck" and "legs," which are then stuck into the apple.

Do-It-Yourself Cranberry Juice

Nutritious and easy to make. Less sweet and mellower than the commercial varieties.

4 cups fresh cranberries
4 cups water
sugar to taste

Cook cranberries in a large pot until they pop and turn translucent. Remove as many berry skins as possible using a slotted spoon. Add sugar to taste and stir well. Cool. Strain as necessary. Pour into juice bottles or pitchers. Refrigerate.

Dried Cranberries

Dried cranberries are similar to raisins, but they're especially appropriate as a festive fall food. Not only are they a good snack for older kids, they're perfect for adding to cold cereal or a muffin batter.

Pumpkin Dessert Cake

If your children aren't big fans of pumpkin pie, this recipe lets you have your traditional pumpkin dessert, but in a form your children will love.

1¼ cups vegetable oil
4 teaspoons vanilla
1 cup honey
1 cup molasses or sugar
4 eggs
2 cups pumpkin or 1 15-ounce can of pumpkin
½ cup wheat germ
2 cups whole-wheat flour
1½ cups white flour
2 teaspoons baking soda
2 tablespoons cinnamon
1 tablespoon nutmeg
1 teaspoon ginger

Combine first six ingredients and mix well. Combine dry ingredients, mix well, then combine with wet ingredients. Mix until blended. Bake at 350°F in two greased bread pans for 1 hour, or in a 9-by-13-inch pan for 35 minutes. Top with Cream-Cheese Frosting. (See page 110.)

Variation: You can make drop cookies from this batter. Bake at 350°F for 10 minutes.

Pumpkin Ice-Cream Pie

1 quart vanilla ice cream
1 15-ounce can pumpkin
½ cup sugar
prepared pie shell (baked) or graham cracker crust
whipped cream (optional)

109

Soften ice cream and mix in pumpkin. Add sugar. Freeze in a prepared crust. Top with whipped cream before serving.

Cream-Cheese Frosting

3–4 ounces cream cheese (either a small package or ½ of the traditional box size)
6 tablespoons butter or margarine
1 teaspoon vanilla
1 tablespoon milk
2 cups powdered sugar

This is a good topping for the Pumpkin Dessert Cake (page 109). Mix ingredients and spread on cooled cake or cookies. Extra frosting makes an excellent filler between two graham crackers.

Peanut-Butter Pinecones

The Peanut-Butter Balls on page 58 can be molded into small pinecone shapes. Poke the narrow ends of sliced almonds (unblanched) into the pinecones at 45° angles in overlapping rows, until the peanut-butter pinecone is covered.

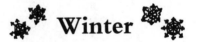

Winter

Take advantage of what's right outside your door—fresh snow! If you find some room in your freezer, pack away clean snow in a plastic bag to use come July for snow cones, recipes, or a mini snowball fight! (*Not advisable in areas with poor air quality.*)

Snow Mousse

2 cups heavy cream
1½ cups powdered sugar
1½ teaspoons vanilla
large bowl of clean, fresh snow

Combine cream, sugar, and vanilla. Whisk in snow gradually, adding more snow until mixture is thick and creamy. Flavorings may be added.

Easy Ice–Cream Snow

1 cup milk
1 pasteurized egg, beaten
½ cup sugar
1 teaspoon vanilla
large bowl of clean, fresh snow

Blend first four ingredients well and add clean, fresh snow until desired consistency is reached.

Orange Snow: Spoon some thawed orange juice concentrate over a dish of snow.

Maple Snow: Pour maple syrup over a dish of snow.

Maple Snow Candy

Fill large pans with fresh, clean, firmly packed snow. Boil real maple syrup until it reaches the soft-ball stage (about 240°F on a candy thermometer), then pour it in a thin stream from a large spoon onto the snow. After the syrup has started to harden, it can be lifted in sections with a fork and twisted into elaborate shapes.

Christmastime

The Christmas holiday is an exciting—and often over-whelming—time of the year. It's a wonderful opportunity for cooking up new and old traditions. Here are some decorating ideas that begin in your kitchen:
• Make cookies to hang on a tree by pushing a plastic straw into a hot cookie just removed from the oven. Twist out a hole at the top of the cookie, removing the straw. Once cooled and hardened, thread a ribbon through the hole and hang from the tree.

- String popcorn after it has been allowed to stand long enough to lose its crispness. Popcorn can also be dyed by dipping it in cranberry juice or other colored beverages.
- Or try stringing mini-marshmallows or colored gumdrops. (Cranberries are too hard for small hands to manage.)
- To add a cheery note to your table, tie bells on a ribbon around a breadbasket.
- Enhance the holiday aroma by adding cinnamon to any play dough you make.

Don't feel you *have* to bake the holiday cookies the kids want to decorate. Buy plain cookies, ready-to-use gels and icing, silver dragées, candied decorations, and colored citrus gummy candies (sliced) that the kids can cut into shapes.

Festive Ideas

- Make "wreath" pancakes and serve with strawberry syrup.
- Serve cooked peas in a scooped-out tomato for its color impact.
- Make a Snack Tree by first covering a conical Styrofoam form with green paper. With toothpicks, attach edibles such as cheese cubes, cherry tomatoes, grapes, cauliflower chunks, green pepper slices, and carrot slices to cover the tree. Serve with a dip.
- Turn homemade cookies into greeting cards by creating larger ones with personal messages written with tube icing.
- Bake bread in a circle or wreath shape. Press in red and green jellybeans for decorations. Add a ribbon bow after bread has cooled.
- Use pointed paper cups for making lime gelatin "trees." Cut away paper when mold is firm, and decorate with cream cheese.
- Create an Orange Sip by rolling an orange between your hands until it's soft. Use a knife to cut an X in the orange. Insert a porous peppermint stick in the X and sip away!

Christmas Trees à la Rice Krispies

You can devise various holiday treats using the well-known Rice Krispies Treats recipe, including these mini Christmas trees.

¼ cup butter or margarine
4 cups mini-marshmallows or 1 6–10 ounce bag
  regular marshmallows
green food coloring
5 cups Rice Krispies
toothpicks
10–12 regular-size marshmallows
red cinnamon candies

Melt butter or margarine in a 3-quart saucepan. Add 4 cups marshmallows and cook over low heat. Stir constantly until syrupy. Remove from heat. Add green food coloring until mixture attains a fairly dark green color. Add cereal and stir until well coated. With buttered hands, shape into conical forms. Cool. Stick a toothpick through a marshmallow and into the bottom of the "tree" to serve as the base. Decorate with red candies.

Variations:
Omit the green food coloring from all the following recipes except Wreaths.

Snowman: Form three balls of mixture in decreasing size. Roll in coconut, stack, and decorate.

Balls: Shape balls of mixture around a nut or date, then roll in colored sugar.

Pops: Shape pops from the mixture in an oval around a Popsicle stick.

Tarts: Press mixture into a buttered muffin tin to form a tart shell. Fill with fresh fruit or ice cream.

113

Wreaths: Shape mixture into a "doughnut." Decorate with red candies.

Gingerbread House

1 gingerbread mix
⅓ cup water
Frosting Cement (page 115)
cardboard
toothpicks

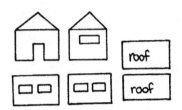

This nifty idea will delight your kids (although not necessarily the nutritionists). Fortunately, it's more to look at than to eat. This simplified recipe does not take a great deal of time.

To one gingerbread mix, add ⅓ cup water. Mix well and roll out into ½-inch thickness. It works best if you take the time to make a cardboard pattern. The base of the house will be about 4-by-6 inches. It will stand about 3½ inches high to the eaves line. You'll need 6 sections.

Cut the door and windows before baking, but do not remove the pieces until after baking. Extra dough can be molded into little cookie people. Bake approximately 15 minutes on a greased sheet for maximum hardness, but do not allow the edges to burn. The house is "glued" together with Frosting Cement. (See page 115.) Use toothpicks wherever necessary. Use the Frosting Cement to hold the base to the plate so it will stand. Let the frame dry before adding the roof.

If this is more than you want to do, just use frosting cement to attach graham crackers to a small milk or orange juice carton. For decoration, add the following:

Snow Landscape: Sprinkle coconut around house, or use cotton.

Roof: Spread with icing and cover with mini-marshmallows, coconut, sprinkles, décors, or candied fruit slices (halved). Or use sections of Shredded Wheat to give a thatched-roof effect. Sliced almonds can look like shingles. Add white icing to a few spots to look like snow on the roof.

Path: Build with small circle candies such as M&Ms, plain chocolate candies, Lifesavers, or sliced gumdrops. Build fences with sugar cubes.

Chimney: Pile 2 or 3 hard circle candies or sugar cubes as a chimney. Cement with frosting.

Trees: Create with green gumdrops, lollipops, pinecones, inverted sugar cones, or tree cookies.

Snowmen: Shape 2 balls from leftover frosting. Let dry. Or stack large marshmallows. Attach with frosting.

Frosting Cement

2 pasteurized egg whites, beaten
½ teaspoon cream of tartar
2 cups powdered sugar

Beat 2 egg whites stiff with ½ teaspoon cream of tartar. Add 2 cups powdered sugar and beat 5 minutes with an electric mixer. Since the mixture dries quickly, keep it covered with a damp cloth when not in use. Makes a smooth, hard-drying icing.

Traditional Gingerbread People

⅔ cup butter or margarine
½ cup sugar
2 teaspoons ginger
1 teaspoon cinnamon
½ teaspoon nutmeg
1 egg
¾ cup molasses
3 cups all-purpose flour, sifted
½ teaspoon baking powder
1 teaspoon baking soda

Put butter or margarine, sugar, spices, and egg in a large mixer bowl. Mix until well blended. Add molasses and mix well. Sift together flour, baking powder, and baking

115

soda. Stir into butter (or margarine) mixture and mix well. Refrigerate at least 2 hours for easier handling.

Roll out on floured board and cut gingerbread-people shapes. Use bits of raisins for eyes, nose, and buttons. Sprinkle with granulated sugar, if desired. Bake on greased baking sheets at 375°F for 8–10 minutes. Makes about a dozen 5-inch gingerbread people.

Hanukkah Hints

- Use Hanukkah cookie cutters on Finger Jell-O (blue-berry and lemon flavors) for appropriate seasonal symbols. (See page 56.)
- Use the Play Clay recipe on pages 131–132 to form festive menorahs.
- Make decorative holiday placemats by drawing with blue crayons on beige or yellow inexpensive vinyl mats.
- For quicker cleanup, spray menorahs with nonstick vegetable spray before placing and lighting candles. (Also good for Kwanzaa candle holders.)

Potato Latkes

Let kids help make the traditional potato latkes each year. Grate 3 peeled potatoes and a bit of onion. Squeeze out excess liquid and drain. Add 2 beaten eggs and 2 table-spoons flour. Heat vegetable oil filled to 1-inch depth in frying pan. Fry small dollops of batter until brown. Turn and cook until crispy. Drain on paper towels and serve with sour cream and/or applesauce.

Valentine's Day

Valentine's Day is a good opportunity to use your heart-shaped cookie cutter on toast, sandwiches, cheese slices, red Finger Jell-O, and, of course, cookies!

Lollipop Heart Cookies

Soak flat wooden Popsicle sticks in cold water for an hour (to keep them from burning when baked with the cookies).

Use the Cuttin' Cookies recipe on pages 101–102. Roll out dough thinly and cut with heart-shaped cookie cutters. Place dough hearts on a baking sheet with at least 2 inches between rows. Place a stick halfway down each heart, making a 2-inch handle. Then place another dough heart on top; press edges and shape gently together. After they've cooled, decorate with white icing or frosting with red décors. Or dip in melted semisweet chocolate chips (letting excess drip back into pan) and cool on wax paper. Add sprinkles or décors before refrigerating to harden.

Valentine Krispies

Use the Rice Krispies Treats recipe on page 113. Add red food coloring to the syrup just before mixing it with the dry cereal. Mold in a greased heart-shaped pan or a greased cookie cutter. Take out and place on a plate to cool.

Need a heart-shaped cake pan but have no such pan? Bake a round and a square layer cake (8-inch or 9-inch) and combine them this way: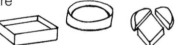

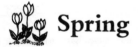 # Spring

The egg is often used symbolically as part of Easter and Passover celebrations. It symbolizes new life in both traditions. An Easter egg hunt (indoors or out) is always great fun. Add some hidden peanuts-in-the-shell to provide extra hunting fun. (*Always keep an accurate tally of how many—and where—eggs are hidden when hiding indoors!*)

Decorating Easter Eggs

Use hard-cooked eggs since they can best take the stress of handling by small children. Take advantage of food-coloring options in your pantry. Let your eggs soak for at least half an hour in bowls of hot water with different colors in each. After removing, let them dry and decorate them with nontoxic magic markers. It's a great medium and easy for kids to handle. An egg carton or a cardboard tube cut into sections makes an excellent drying and decorating stand. When finished, put a drop of butter or margarine on your hands and rub over each egg to give it a shine and to set the color. You can also glue on additions such as ribbon, rickrack, and even plastic "eyes." Serve decorated hard-cooked eggs throughout the Easter season.

Variation: Decorate using washable markers, paints, or gel pens.

Egg-Shaped Cookies

Make an egg-shaped cookie cutter by bending and shaping the open end of a 6-ounce juice can. Decorate with a variety of icings or with Egg-Yolk Paint. (See recipe below.) If you're not up to making your own dough, use a roll of refrigerated sugar cookies and shape.

Egg-Yolk Paint

Blend ¼ teaspoon water with 1 pasteurized egg yolk. Divide among several small dishes and put different food coloring in each dish. Paint designs on cookies before baking.

Jell-O Eggs

With a small nail, poke a hole in the narrow end of an empty plastic egg (the kind that comes apart). Wash the egg, wipe the inside with a little vegetable oil, and put the two halves together. Fill with Finger Jell-O (page 56) and set upright until Jell-O is firm. Remove shell after Jell-O has hardened. Regular Jell-O can also be used here, but use half of the cold water called for.

Also, you can turn any Finger Jell-O recipe into pastel colors by dissolving 2 4-ounce packages of gelatin in 1 cup of boiling water. After it cools to room temperature, whip in 8 ounces of Cool Whip (in place of additional water) and combine with 6 ounces of Jell-O dissolved in

1 cup boiling water. After firmed up in the refrigerator, use bunny or egg-shaped cookie cutters to create pastel treats.

Egg Tree

A branch can be decorated attractively using decorated eggshells. Here you must blow out the inside of the raw egg before decorating and hanging it. Use glue to affix strings. If a budding branch is put in a narrow-necked vase with water, leaves will soon adorn the branch along with the decorated eggs.

Bunny Salad

Place a canned pear half on a bed of lettuce. Add raisins for eyes, a strawberry (with a toothpick) for the nose, toothpicks for whiskers, and thin-sliced cheese (or paper) for the ears. Or, using your favorite egg salad recipe, shape serving into a bunny shape.

Bunny Biscuits

Use refrigerated biscuits. Cut one in half horizontally, then cut one of those pieces in half to use as the head. Cut the remaining piece in half for the ears. Pinch out a bit for the tail and bake as directed.

Bunny Ice-Cream Dish

Arrange 3 balls of vanilla ice cream on a plate to form a bunny. Use a large one for the body, a medium one for the head, and a small one for the tail. Cover with shredded coconut. Use jellybeans or almonds for the eyes and nose, paper cutouts for the ears, and toothpicks or licorice string for whiskers.

Bunny Cakes

Version One: Bake a cake in a heart-shaped pan and cover it with white or pink frosting. Decorate it as shown in the diagram, using paper cutouts for ears, jellybeans for eyes and nose, and icing or licorice string for whiskers.

Version Two: Bake cake in a one-layer cake pan. Cut layer in half, as shown. Stand 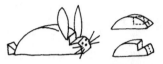 layers side by side, attaching them with a filling of your choice. Shape rabbit by cutting out notch to make a body and head. Use notch for tail. Frost with fluffy white frosting and sprinkle with coconut. Insert paper ears, jellybeans for eyes and nose, and licorice strings for whiskers. Sprinkle green-tinted coconut and more jellybeans on the cake platter.

Tinted Coconut: Add a few drops of food coloring to a small amount of water in a bowl. Add coconut and toss with a fork until evenly distributed. Or, in a small jar, toss 1½ cups coconut with 1–2 tablespoons fruit-flavored Jell-O. Shake well.

Easter Baskets

- Use a pipe cleaner as a handle on a margarine tub. Fill with seedless green grapes.
- Decorate a frosted cupcake with green-tinted coconut. Use pipe cleaners to form the basket handle.
- Weave ribbons in and out of green, plastic berry baskets, and add a handle and some plastic "grass" for a quick, colorful basket.
- Turn a third of the bottom part of an egg carton into a decorative egg holder. Paint the section and add a handle (using pipe cleaners) with a bow so kids can easily carry four eggs safely.

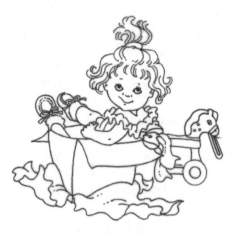

Chapter Seven
So You're Having a Birthday Party!

Here are a few insights to help you make your child's birthday party the happy time it's supposed to be:
- Plan ahead.
- Keep it short and simple.
- Keep it moving.
- Don't invite more children than the number of years in your child's age.

Keep in mind that young children enjoy most what they know best. This is not the age for surprise parties. Build on tradition. Offer the same songs, cakes, balloons, candles, gifts, and games that have always been favorites. For more party ideas for these ages, see Vicki Lansky's *Birthday Parties: Best Party Tips & Ideas* (Book Peddlers).

Year One

This party is really for adults—grandparents, aunts and uncles, cousins, a favorite babysitter, a neighbor or two, or close friends. Keep the guest list small. The food can be fancy and adult-oriented because your baby will care very little about it, unless he or she can get hands into the goo or ice cream. Your child will be bewildered by the presents but will truly enjoy the attention, excitement, and picture taking.

If your plans include other small children, consider a BYOHC (bring your own highchair) party. Provide disposable bibs, travel packages of baby wipes, and teething biscuits as favors. Have your camera ready, too. There's only one first birthday party! Limit the party to an hour.

Year Two

By the second year, the miracle of maturation gives your child a clear understanding of a birthday party, its food, and its presents. Keep the party as small—yes, as small—as possible. Two-year-olds are a bit young for games yet. A supply of toys and balloons works well. Since sharing is not usually a strong point at this age, you may spend some time refereeing. Odds are you'll also be entertaining the mommies and possibly the daddies.

A good food idea for the children is something simple like cupcakes and/or ice-cream cones with sprinkles. Disposable bibs and baby wipes may still be in order. The birthday cake with the candles may be for the adults, but only after its candles are blown out and the children are served their share. Don't waste good food on the kids—they usually don't eat more than a few bites. Limit the party to an hour or an hour and a half.

Year Three

Now you're entering the realm of the more traditional birthday party. Games can be played and enjoyed, although they must definitely be led. Keep it simple. Three to five short games should suffice. Avoid competitive games unless everyone can get a prize. A quiet game or storytelling is a better prelude to refreshments than active games. (See the list of games at the end of this chapter.)

Your three-year-old is beginning to learn social graces. Manners won't be perfect, but this can be a good starting point. Greeting guests, opening presents, expressing thanks, and saying good-bye are behaviors to be discussed before the party and praised afterward.

Your child should also be consulted about the guest list. He or she can help mail or deliver invitations and help choose and/or frost the cake. Written thanks for presents are not necessary.

Food should again be simple. If you're dying to try an unusual form of cake, don't. Children do enjoy form cakes; just don't get carried away. Three-year-olds judge most cakes by their icing alone.

Also save yourself time and hassle by scooping out ice-cream balls ahead of time. Place them in cupcake papers and store in the freezer until you're ready for them. Or buy ice-cream cups and serve them with their wooden spoons.

A fun place card is a cookie with each child's name written on it in icing. Or let each child decorate his or her own cookie. Provide icing, a Popsicle stick, and decorations such as sprinkles, nuts, raisins, chocolate chips, and coconut.

Do include a "hunt" (for candy, peanuts, or other prizes) in your party. A party hat or small plastic bag is an appropriate holder. Save some extra goodies in case any child totally misses the boat.

While candy is an integral part of any party, you may want to include more nutritious treats. Consider these:

- Chocolate- or yogurt-covered raisins
- Finger Jell-O (page 56)
- Fruit Roll (pages 61–62)
- Peanuts-in-the-shell
- Pretzels tied with ribbons
- Raisins, nuts, and sunflower seeds
- Sugarless bubble gum
- Uncandy Bars (pages 59–60)

A favorite treat that makes a birthday special is Candy Cookies. (See below.) Bake them for a party either at home or at preschool. If you add the candies to the cookie tops and use the Cornell Triple-Rich Formula (page 84), you'll strike a compromise between the kids' love for candy and their need for a bit of nutrition. Limit the party to an hour and a half.

Candy Cookies

1 cup vegetable oil
1 cup brown sugar, packed
½ cup sugar
2 eggs
2 teaspoons vanilla
1½ teaspoons baking soda
2¼ cups flour (See Cornell Triple-Rich Formula on page 84.)
1 cup (or less) plain M&Ms

Cream oil, sugars, eggs, and vanilla. Mix dry ingredients and combine with creamed mixture. Drop by teaspoonfuls on an ungreased baking sheet. Flatten to not more than a 2-inch diameter. Decorate with 4–6 candies per cookie. (To avoid hassles, make sure the number is the same for every cookie.) Bake at 375°F for 8–10 minutes. The candies often crack after baking. This recipe makes 2–4 dozen cookies, depending on the size of your teaspoonful.

We can offer no advice on presents, prizes, or party favors. You alone must live with your budget and your neighbors. But remember, *more* does not mean *better*.

Year Four

Most of what goes for a three-year-old's party is applicable here—and more so. By now, the moms and dads are no longer on the sidelines to help, so it's up to you to keep the ball rolling. If it's too much for you to be leader, song director, photographer, server, and cleanup committee, have someone help you—possibly a neighborhood teenager.

While you're waiting for all the guests to arrive, alleviate any awkwardness by having a planned activity. String a birthday necklace, decorate a favor bag, or even open presents.

Four-year-olds anticipate games eagerly. A variety of *short* games is good for their short attention spans. (See the list at the end of this chapter.) In addition to games, a clown or puppet show would be a treat. Check on the talents of some of the older children in your neighborhood, or look at the ads in your area's parenting newspaper or tabloid magazine.

You may find yourself holding the party around lunch or dinnertime. Here are foods with the best chance of being eaten:

- Grilled cheese sandwiches
- Pizza
- Macaroni and cheese
- Hamburgers
- Peanut-butter-and-jelly sandwiches (cut with a cookie cutter)
- Potato chips (Individual bags are a treat.)
- Carrot sticks
- Dill pickles
- Apple wedges
- Mandarin oranges
- Green grapes (seedless)
- Juice (apple, pineapple, orange)
- Chocolate milk

Sandwiches should be "crustless!" After all, this is a party. Avoid drinks that stain. Juice boxes (or pouches) are special as well as spill-proof. Make food portions small. Children often eat very little because they're too excited.

For a different ice-cream treat, cut off the tops of oranges and scoop out the insides. Put in orange sherbet and freeze until ready to serve. Consider do-it-yourself sundaes, letting children help themselves to their favorite ice-cream toppings including fudge, honey, maple syrup, granola, nuts, crushed pineapple, coconut, and whipped cream. Or make clown cones. Top a scoop of ice cream with a

125

sugar cone for a hat and create a face on it. Reddi-wip makes good "hair." Make ahead of time and freeze.

Don't feel you have to seat a group of children in your dining room. Any appropriate room with a vinyl tablecloth on the floor and low tables (coffee table, card tables on books, or bricks) will work just fine. While you can specify a pickup time, returning your guests to their homes lets you end the party on *your* schedule. Limit the party to two hours.

Year Five

While home parties for this age are still recommended, away-from-home parties will also work. Avoid movies but check out gymnastics programs, skating rinks, hamburger franchises, pizza parlors, ice-cream parlors, and even your local zoo.

Birthday Party Dangers

Beware of:
- Little children with long hair trying to blow out candles. (Hair burns.)
- Children running with straws or lollipops in their mouths.
- Children playing with (and choking on) uninflated or broken balloons.

Preschool Games

Let your birthday child be the first to be *it* in a game. Plan more games than you think you'll need in case some turn out to be too hard or unpopular. On the other hand, don't feel you must play all the games you planned—or ones the birthday child doesn't like or isn't good at. The younger the guests, the more likely you'll have some who don't want to play every game. So have alternative activities available, such as coloring books or puzzles.

The following games are recommended for ages two to five. They're listed from simpler to more complex.

- *Ball Roll:* Children roll a ball to each other while sitting in a circle with legs spread.
- *Tell a Story:* An adult reads a book with large pictures or makes up a story. Keep it short.
- *Action Songs:* Examples include "Ring around the Rosy," "Farmer in the Dell," "London Bridge," "Eensy Weensy Spider," and "Hokey Pokey."
- *Animal Parade:* Children march around imitating elephants, bunnies, dogs, cats, birds, kangaroos, or other animals.
- *Pin the Tail on the Donkey:* Or pin the nose on the clown.
- *Drop (or Toss) a Beanbag into a Basket.*
- *Simple Simon:* Keep it simple!
- *Balloon Push:* Outdoors, it can be done by kicking; indoors by crawling and using one's nose.
- *Kangaroo Race:* Children hop while holding a balloon between their knees.
- *Ring the Bell:* Hang a bell in a tree outside or in a doorway inside. Children throw a beanbag or Nerf ball at the bell, which rings when hit.
- *Musical Chairs:* Play the way you remember it, or adopt a variation such as passing a plastic or tin plate. The holder when the music stops is "out."
- *Dress Up:* Have a large pile of oversized clothes, hats, and shoes that kids can race to get into simultaneously. (Take photos.)
- *Duck, Duck, Gray Duck (a.k.a. Duck, Duck, Goose):* A circle game of tag.
- *Doggie, Doggie, Who's Got the Bone?:* Children sit in a circle around a blindfolded child sitting in the center. An object is given to one of the outer children. The children put their hands behind their backs and say, "Doggie, Doggie, where's your bone? Someone has taken it far from home!" The child in the center takes the blindfold off and is given three chances to guess who has the "bone."

127

- *Shoe Race:* Children remove their shoes and place them in a pile. When they get the signal, they hurry to find and put on their shoes (without buckling, fastening, or tying) and race to the finish line.
- *Bingo!*

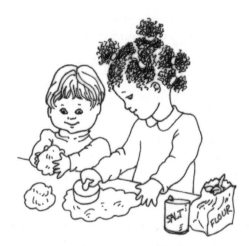

Chapter Eight
Kitchen Crafts

Your time is often spent in your kitchen—and your child's is, too—so give your child a chance to do some creative "messing around"! Many grown-up jobs can be shared with youngsters. Don't expect perfection. Remember, they're new to these tasks.

- Washing dishes, dirty or not
- Setting the table
- Folding napkins
- Washing and cleaning vegetables
- Scrubbing the floor
- Cleaning the kitchen sink (It'll be spotless—in some spots!)

Doughs, Clays, and Pastes

If you've never made your own modeling clay, now's the time to start. Here are three recipes, each with special characteristics. Experiment to find your favorite. (Your child's age may determine the best one to use.) When using any form of modeling clay, don't neglect the necessary equipment including cookie cutters, rolling pins (real or play), plastic knives, bottle caps, extra flour, uncooked spaghetti or macaroni, walnut half shells, and others—limited only by your and your child's imaginations.

No–Cook Play Dough

1 cup white flour
½ cup salt
2 tablespoons vegetable oil
1 teaspoon alum
food coloring
½ cup water

Mix first four ingredients. Add food coloring to the water. Gradually add small amounts of water until mixture attains the consistency of bread dough. You may not use the entire ½ cup of water. You can make colors that are not commercially available, such as purple, by creatively mixing colors. Store in an airtight container or plastic bag. It lasts a long time. (If you can't find alum in the grocery store, look in the drugstore.)

Stove–Top Play Dough

1 cup white flour
¼ cup salt
2 tablespoons cream of tartar
1 cup water
1 teaspoon food coloring
1 tablespoon vegetable oil

Mix flour, salt, and cream of tartar in a medium-size pot. Add water, food coloring, and oil. Cook and stir over medium heat for 3–5 minutes. Mixture will look like a globby mess, and you'll be sure it's not turning out, but it will. When it forms a ball in the center of the pot, turn out and knead on a lightly floured surface. Store in an airtight container or plastic bag. Edible but not as tasty as Play Dough à la Peanut Butter! (See page 131.)

Play Dough à la Peanut Butter

1 18-ounce jar peanut butter
6 tablespoons honey
cocoa or carob (optional)
nonfat dry milk or milk plus flour, to the right consistency

Mix all ingredients. After shaping, decorate (try raisins) and eat!

Variation: Mix 1 can of frosting, 1½ cups powdered sugar, and 1 cup peanut butter. When your child is old enough to appreciate something a bit more permanent, add "real" homemade clay to your bag of tricks.

Clay for Play and Posterity

Baking Method:

1 cup salt
½ cup water
2 tablespoons vegetable oil
2 cups flour

Mix salt, water, and oil. Add flour. After shaping, clay can be baked at 250°F for several hours.

Overnight Drying Method:

1 cup cornstarch
2 cups baking soda (1 pound)
1¼ cups cold water
food coloring, tempera, or acrylic paints (optional)
shellac or clear nail polish (optional)

Mix cornstarch, baking soda, and water. Stir in a saucepan over medium heat for about 4 minutes until mixture thickens to the consistency of moist mashed potatoes. Remove from heat, turn out on a plate, and cover with a damp cloth until cool. Knead as you would bread dough. Shape as desired or store in an airtight container or plastic bag.

To color, add a few drops of food coloring to the water before mixing it with starch and soda. Or leave objects to dry and then paint with tempera or acrylics. Dip in shellac or brush with clear nail polish to seal.

Clay Christmas Ornaments
(Oven Drying Method)

4 cups flour
1 cup salt
1 teaspoon alum
1½ cups water
food coloring, poster paints, acrylic paints, or markers
clear shellac, spray plastic, or nail polish

Mix first four ingredients well in a large bowl. If the dough is too dry, work in another tablespoon of water with your hands. Dough can be colored by dividing it into several parts and kneading a drop or two of food coloring into each part. Roll or mold as desired. (If you can't find alum in the grocery store, look in the drugstore.)

To Roll: Roll dough ⅛-inch thick on lightly floured board. Cut with cookie cutters dipped in flour. Make a hole in the top, ¼-inch from the edge, with the end of a plastic straw dipped in flour. Shake the dot of clay from the straw and press on as decoration. Thread ribbon or wire through the hole to hang ornament.

To Mold: Shape dough into figures (such as flowers, fruits, and animals) no more than ½-inch thick. Insert a fine wire in each for hanging.

Bake ornaments at 250°F on an ungreased baking sheet for about 30 minutes. Turn ornaments over and bake another 1½ hours until hard and dry. Remove and cool. When done, sand lightly with fine sandpaper until smooth. Paint with food coloring, plastic-based poster paint, acrylic paint, or markers. Paint both sides. Allow paint to dry and seal with clear shellac, spray plastic, or clear nail polish. Makes about 5 dozen 2½-inch ornaments.

Clay Cookie Ornaments (Overnight Drying Method)

2 cups salt
⅔ cup water
1 cup (or more) cornstarch
½ cup cold water

Mix salt with ⅔ cup water and boil. Add cornstarch and remaining water. Stir. If mixture doesn't thicken, set back on stove. Sprinkle extra cornstarch on table and rolling pin. Roll out dough and cut with cookie cutters. Use a plastic straw to make a hole at the top for hanging. Let dry. Use paint, glitter, and so on to decorate. *These are not edible!*

Bread Clay Recipe

6 slices white bread
6 tablespoons white glue
1 teaspoon white vinegar
½ teaspoon detergent or 2 teaspoons glycerin
food coloring

Who said plain white bread is worthless? Remove crusts and knead bread with white glue, vinegar, and detergent or glycerin. Knead mixture until it becomes nonsticky. Separate into portions and tint each with food coloring. Shape and, when done, brush with equal parts glue and water for a smooth appearance. Let dry overnight to harden. Acrylic paints, spray plastic, or clear nail polish will seal and preserve your child's art "treasures."

Homemade Silly Putty/Gak-Like Goo

2 parts Elmer's white glue
1 part Sta-Flo Regular Liquid Starch

Mix well. Putty must dry a bit before it's workable. It may be necessary to add a bit more glue or starch; you'll have to experiment. Some suggest equal parts; others have success with a starch-to-glue ratio of 2 to 1. (*Recipe may not work well on a humid day.*) Store in an airtight container. Beware of contact with clothes and carpet. If you use Elmer's school glue instead of regular white glue, it doesn't bounce or pick up pictures, but it makes a gooey delight your kids will love. Use on a smooth surface. Store in a Ziploc bag.

Alternative: In a glass bowl, mix 1 container (4 ounces or ⅓ cup) Elmer's White Glue-All (not school glue), ⅓ cup water, and 6 drops food coloring. Fill a liquid measuring cup with ⅓ cup water. Add 3–4 tablespoons of borax and stir. Pour off excess water so only wet borax remains. Add to glue-water mixture. A solid blob will grow as you mix it in. Place this lump on wax paper and knead. Wetness will disappear as you work it. Add extra glue-water mixture to the now solid "putty" as needed. Store in a plastic bag.

Hint: Use WD-40 to remove commercial Silly Putty from carpet. Then blot with rubbing alcohol until stain is gone.

No-Cook Paste

water
handful of flour
pinch of salt

Gradually add water to flour and mix until gooey. Add salt. This recipe can also be used as a quickie finger paint by adding some food coloring and working it on heavy paper or cardboard. Also works well as a papier-mâché paste.

Library Paste

1 cup flour
1 cup sugar

1 teaspoon alum
4 cups water
oil of cloves or wintergreen

Mix first four ingredients in a saucepan. Cook until clear and thick. Add 30 drops of oil of cloves or wintergreen. Store in a covered container. (If you can't find alum in the grocery store, look in the drugstore.)

Glass Glue

2 packets unflavored gelatin
2 tablespoons cold water
3 tablespoons skim milk

Soften gelatin in cold water in a bowl. Heat milk to boiling and add to softened gelatin. Stir until gelatin dissolves. Pour into a jar. Use this when something must adhere to glass, such as labels on jars, or to glue wood to wood. Keeps only a day or two. Set jar in a pan of hot water to soften for reuse.

Lightweight Glue

Egg white makes a good adhesive for constructing kites. It's strong and almost weightless. Liquid starch or corn syrup work as glue for many projects, especially facial decorations at Halloween. It allows cotton or oatmeal to adhere to kids' faces.

Finger Paints

Finger painting doesn't occupy the attention of small children for as long as parents would like, and cleanup always seems to take longer than play time. But it's worth the effort for the discovery and fun. Don't show your child how to use finger paints as you think they should be used—experimenting is the best part for your child. Sometimes it's fun just to feel the cool, smooth paint and see the bright colors. A linoleum floor covered with newspapers is often the best painting location since the floor often has to be cleaned after a painting session anyway! Powdered poster paint is still a good investment when you do a lot of water-based-paint activities. It lasts a long time and can be found in art-supply stores, craft stores, and teacher stores.

#1 Finger Paints

3 tablespoons sugar
½ cup cornstarch
2 cups cold water
food coloring
pinch of detergent

Mix the sugar and cornstarch, then add water. Cook over low heat, stirring constantly until well blended. Divide mixture into four or five portions and add a different food coloring to each, plus a pinch of detergent to facilitate cleanup.

#2 Finger Paints

½ cup dry laundry starch
¼ cup cold water
1½ cups boiling water
½ cup soap flakes
1 teaspoon glycerin
food coloring

Mix starch and cold water in a saucepan. Pour in boiling water and cook over low heat until shiny. Remove from heat and add soap and glycerin. Divide into portions and add different food coloring.

Soapy Finger Paints

Add a drop of food coloring or paint to aerosol shaving cream, and let your child do his or her thing on a baking sheet. If you don't want to go to the trouble of mixing finger paints, squirt the cream on a baking sheet and add the color to it.

Canned Kid Paint

For quickie finger paints, just add food coloring to sweetened condensed milk that you've divided into different small bowls.

Brushes

- Try a pastry brush if you can spare yours. They have wider handles, and the stiffer brush cuts down on splatters.
- Or try cotton swabs. A different swab can be used for each color so the paints (hopefully) remain unmixed and bright.

Face Paint

Mix one part solid shortening (like Crisco) to two parts cornstarch. Add food coloring for desired effects. Add enough glycerin to allow the paint to spread smoothly on the skin.

Printing

Printing—Vegetable Style

Cut a potato, carrot, or turnip in half and carve out a raised design (Mom or Dad's job). Brush poster paints over the design, or stamp the design in an ink pad. Press firmly on paper (white tissue paper, uncoated shelf paper, ribbons, or anything you have around). Let dry. Sliced citrus fruits, apples, and onions also make lovely prints.

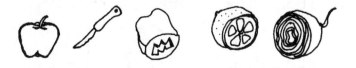

Printing Utensils

While sponges (plain or cut into shapes) are the most obvious printing utensils, also try a potato masher, a wooden salad fork, bottoms of extract bottles, and toothbrushes.

Paper Product Paraphernalia

Here are just a few ideas for using everyday items.

Straws

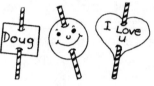

To make any day special, and perhaps to encourage drinking a disliked beverage, try this trick. Make a cutout in a circle or a special shape. (One paper plate will provide several cutouts.) Use a hole puncher to make a hole in the top and bottom of your cutout. Decorate the cutout, or let your child do so, then weave a straw in one hole and out the other. (If you include names on your cutouts, these could be dandy place cards for a birthday party.)

Paper Plates

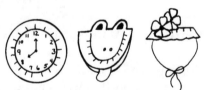

These can be made into clocks, puppets, or hats.

Milk Cartons

There are many things you can do with empty milk cartons. One fun idea is to make building blocks. Use two milk cartons of the same size. Open the top ends completely, then slide the cartons together (as shown) to make a block. Cover with Contact paper to decorate.

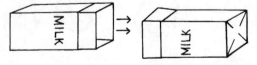

Paper Cups

These can be made into:

Bells: Decorate.

Minidrum: Cover top with paper and hold in place with a rubber band.

Telephone: Connect two cups with a long string.

Spyglasses: Attach two cups side-by-side with tape. Punch holes in the bottoms for eyes, and use string to secure around the head.

Brown Paper Bags

- Large brown paper bags make good life-size masks and costumes for young children. Help children cut out facial features and holes for arms, but let them do the rest.
- To make a flashlight face, cut out facial features on the base of a paper bag. Insert the head of the flashlight into the top of the bag. Twist the bag around the flashlight (leaving the switch exposed) and fasten with tape or string.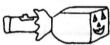
- A small brown bag makes an excellent hand puppet. (Make the "head" on the base of the bag.)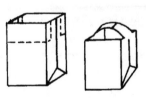
- Or make a tote bag as shown:
- Paper bags that have been decorated (but not cut into) can later be used as garbage or recycling bags.
- For a great collection of ideas on how to use bags, check out Vicki Lansky's *The Bag Book* (Book Peddlers).

Miscellaneous Fun

Stained-Glass Crayons

A good way to use all those broken crayon pieces
(which always seem to be in abundant supply) is to
make stained-glass crayons. Remove any covering
paper, place the pieces in a well-greased muffin tin (or
line each muffin section with tin foil), and put in a 400°F
oven for a few minutes until melted. Remove from the
oven and cool completely before removing from tin. If
you mix the crayon colors, these crayon circles will have
a lovely stained-glass effect and are great fun to color with.

Peanut-Butter Bird Feeder

Spread peanut butter on each "leaf" of a pinecone. Roll
in a dish of birdseed. Using a piece of yarn or wire, hang
it from a tree.

Rainbow Celery

Place a cut stalk of celery with leaves still on it in a glass
of water tinted with food coloring. Within an hour the
color begins to show in the leaves. Slice one stalk in half
part way up from the bottom and place each stem in
separate glasses of differently colored water for a
multicolored effect.

Chase the Pepper

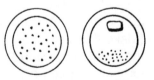

You don't have to understand
the scientific principle to be
entertained by this magic trick. Fill a pie plate (or a small
sink) with water. Shake pepper on the water. Take a
piece of wet soap and dip it into the water. The pepper
will run away from the soap. Now shake some sugar into
the clear area and the pepper will run back.

The Classic Rubber Egg

Every child should experience (at least once) the disgusting "rubber egg" experiment. Place an uncooked egg (in its shell) in a glass jar and pour white vinegar over it until covered. Leave for at least two days, then pour off the vinegar. You'll now have a yucky-to-the-touch but fascinating egg object. It's perfect for a Halloween haunted-house experience. Let kids touch it blindfolded, and say it's a human eye.

Crystal Garden

4 tablespoons salt (not iodized)
4 tablespoons water
4 tablespoons ammonia
4 tablespoons liquid wash bluing

Mix ingredients. Pour over several small pieces of charcoal, sponge, or crumbled cork in a bowl. Put several drops of different-colored inks or food coloring on various parts. Leave undisturbed for a day. Crystals will cover the pieces in an interesting formation, growing and spreading every day. Pieces will be white where no coloring was used. (The garden grows better in dry air than humid air.)

How Does Your Garden Grow?

There are several easily grown items that may be of special wintertime delight to your child. He or she can do all the work. A good functional container is a cut-down milk carton filled with potting soil, with holes punched in the bottom for drainage. Or you may want to use an eggshell half. Three-quarters of an eggshell, decorated, makes a delightful pot. Better yet, the shell can be a "head" with green, growing "hair." Place the "pot" in a sunny or well-lit window.

Avocados: Though the avocado pit is a popular item to grow, it's not very exciting for small children since germination is often very slow.

Cress: Most types of cress are easy to grow and can be added to salads a few weeks after planting.

Dried beans: Roll a piece of paper towel in a clear glass. Put a lima bean, corn kernel, or other dried bean between the paper and the side of the glass. Keep the paper moist. You can watch the seed send roots down and sprouts up.

Citrus seeds: Place 4 or 5 seeds (orange, lemon, or grapefruit) in a container and cover with ½ inch of soil. Keep soil moist by gently covering with clear wrap until the seeds have germinated.

Sweet potatoes: Place a large sweet potato in a shallow dish with enough water to cover it. Keep it half-covered in water as the days pass. It will grow a lovely vine for you. If you have no luck, try a new potato, since sweet potatoes are often treated to prevent growth.

Carrots: Cut the green top from a carrot. Place the top in a few inches of water. The top will sprout again.

Grass seed or birdseed: Place on a wet sponge in a shallow dish. A little water should always show above the sponge, so you know it hasn't dried out. Eventually your child can "mow the lawn" if he or she can handle a scissors.

Chapter Nine
Parent Potpourri
(Or, "I Wish I'd Thought of That!")

This final chapter is a collection of everything that didn't fit anywhere else. It contains many useful ideas passed along from "practicing" parents to new parents—practical information collected in one place for your reference.

Busy Little People Make Spots

Here are some tried-and-true methods for removing spots that are sure to show up as your child grows:

- *Milk spots on upholstery or carpet:* Rub in baking soda and vacuum. Baking soda will prevent stains and odors. Window cleaner spray or baby wipes are often effective for other stains.
- *Bloodstains:* Rinse in cold water. Then soak in cold water with salt before washing as usual. Or let hydrogen peroxide bubble through the fabric to help release the stain before washing.
- *Urine on a rug:* This requires fast action. Keep the following solution on hand for a prompt response: ½ cup

vinegar mixed with ¾ cup water. Apply small amounts to the stain. Give the solution a few minutes to work and then sponge from the outside to the center. Blot dry with a cloth. Another recommended solution is to sprinkle baking soda on the area, then add water and blot dry with a cloth or paper towel.

- *Marks on appliances and windows:* Mix ¼ cup alcohol, 1 tablespoon white vinegar, and 1 tablespoon non-sudsy ammonia. Add enough hot water to make one quart. Cleans without film or streaks.

Baby Cleanup

- *Baby bottles and toys:* A few spoonfuls of baking soda in a quart of water cleans baby bottles and toys and freshens a diaper bag and plastic diaper covers. Add baking soda to your diaper pail to minimize odors.
- *Baby's silver gifts:* Rub a small amount of toothpaste over them with a damp cloth, then rinse clean.
- *After-meal mess:* After-meal "swabbing" is seldom appreciated by babies. You can ease the task by applying petroleum jelly or baby oil to your baby's chin and cheeks before a meal. A warm washcloth or soft baby washcloth will probably be met with less resistance. Play peek-a-boo with the washcloth, cleaning a little each time. Most of the food will be removed—and so will the hassle. You can also put a small bowl of water on the highchair tray for your child to play with after a meal. All you need to do is wipe clean hands dry! When your little one is old enough, give him or her a damp washcloth or puppet washcloth for self-cleanup. A dab of toothpaste spread over an upper-lip stain removes it quickly.
- *Highchair cleanup:* In warm weather, take it outside and hose it down. Otherwise, give it a shower in your shower.

Toddler Cleanup

- *Crayon marks:* Remove from vinyl tile or linoleum with silver polish. To remove from woodwork, rub lightly with a dry, soap-filled steel-wool pad. On blackboards or cabinets, use baking soda on a damp sponge.

- *Dirty white socks:* Boil in water with a slice of lemon. Or soak in hot water in the washing machine for half an hour using ½ cup dishwasher detergent. If socks are cotton, add 1 cup chlorine bleach. If they're a blend, use a nonchlorine whitener.
- *Ballpoint ink on fabrics:* Spray hairspray directly on the stain and wipe away with warm, sudsy water. It's the alcohol that makes it work.
- *Bubble gum in hair:* Peanut butter is a terrific remedy. (Then you're just stuck with washing out the peanut butter!) Solid shortening (like Crisco) or cold cream is also effective. To remove bubble gum from fabric, cover the area with a piece of wax paper and run a warm iron over the wax paper quickly until the gum dissolves.
- *Stuffed toys:* Clean by rubbing with cornstarch. Let stand briefly, then brush off.
- *Finger marks on wallpaper:* Rub chunks of soft, stale bread over the wallpaper to remove.
- *Velcro losing its stick?* Run a stiff toothbrush, pen, or fine-toothed metal comb through the rough side.

Don't forget to keep those handy stain sticks in your diaper bag, near your changing area, and near the washing machine. (*But remember, they're not for a little one to play with*!)

Parent on Duty

Parenthood, you'll quickly discover, is an on-the-job training program. Keep in mind that feeding schedules usually disappear during illnesses. Even a minor illness usually means that foods give way to liquids. Give your child plenty to drink if your child isn't vomiting. Your child's appetite will make up for lost meals when good health returns.

Your doctor may recommend a clear-liquid diet including Fruit Ice (see page 146), Popsicles, frozen orange juice on a stick, Kool-Aid, clear broth, Jell-O, fruit punches, and soft drinks such as 7-UP or ginger ale that have been allowed to go flat. If your child won't drink the needed liquids from a cup, offer a straw when he or she is in the bathtub.

Fruit Ice or Popsicles are excellent first-aid measures for cut lips and bumped mouths. They slow the bleeding, reduce swelling, numb the area, and take your child's mind off the discomfort.

Fruit Ice

finely crushed ice
frozen juice concentrate, thawed

Place ice in a cup and pour juice over it. Drink or eat with a spoon (as a snow cone).

First-Aid Tips

- Give a child liquid medicine in a nipple, eyedropper, or syringe dispenser you can buy at the drugstore. (*Don't give medications in the dark.*)
- Honey and lemon juice make a good homemade cough syrup. (*Don't give to babies under one year of age.*)
- A small hair curler makes a good "cast" for a bruised finger. A wooden Popsicle stick can be used as a splint.
- An ice cube will help numb an area when you need to remove a splinter.
- Use a frozen juice can or bag of frozen vegetables as a quick, dripless compress. Or keep a Ziploc plastic bag filled with half water, half rubbing alcohol in your freezer. It will conform to different shapes. Refreeze and use as needed.
- When removing an adhesive bandage, rub it first with baby oil to make it "ouchless."
- A pill is swallowed more easily in a teaspoon of apple-sauce or yogurt.
- Give liquid vitamins or medicines during bath time to avoid stains on clothes.

- Treat a bee sting quickly with a paste of baking soda and water. Or use meat tenderizer and water. Ice can help numb the area.
- For diaper rash, cautiously use a hair dryer set on cool (at a safe distance) to dry a sore bottom between diaper changes. Fresh air, in any form, is the best treatment for a rampant rash. Solid vegetable shortening can be used as a moisture-barrier ointment.
- Immediate treatment for a burn is cold water. For a larger burn (including sunburn), cover the area with a cold, wet towel.
- Warm a wet compress in your slow cooker, or put it in the microwave for 10 seconds.

Feeding Guidelines When Your Child Is Ill

Sore Throat

Offer soothing suckers such as lollipops, Popsicles, frozen orange juice on a stick, ice cream, and ice chips.

Fever

Give liquids in whatever form your child will accept. If your child won't drink large amounts, try small amounts at frequent intervals. Sometimes your child will drink more by going back to a bottle. Check with your doctor before giving acetaminophen or ibuprofen.

Vomiting

Forget food. Wait a little while before giving your child small sips of liquid. To assure a slow intake, let your child suck on an ice cube or crushed ice. Continue giving small amounts of liquid in gradually increasing intervals until you're sure your child's stomach is settled. If your child vomits the liquid, wait an hour or two before trying again.

Appropriate liquids include decarbonated sodas such as 7 UP or ginger ale, weak tea, "Jell-O Water" (1 package Jell-O and 1 quart water), and commercial rehydrating solutions such as Pedialyte, which comes in several flavors and is good for replacing fluids and electrolytes. Older children may prefer a sports drink such as Gatorade. Once your child hasn't vomited for several hours, begin easy solids such as crackers or plain toast. If vomiting recurs, start from the top. Check with your doctor if vomiting continues for more than six hours.

Diarrhea

Check with your doctor if your baby is under six months of age. Continue breastfeeding. For toddlers or preschoolers, discontinue cow's milk until symptoms disappear. Serve appropriate liquids at room temperature, including juices, decarbonated sodas, Pedialyte, weak tea, "Jell-O Water" (in this case, 1 package Jell-O and 1 cup water), and carrot soup (made by mixing 1 jar of commercial strained carrots with 1 jar water). Give Gatorade to older children to replace lost minerals and fluids.

Easy, binding solids include mashed potatoes, rice cereal, Jell-O, dry toast, crackers, bananas, and applesauce. A common way to remember these is the BRAT diet:

Bananas
Rice cereal
Applesauce
Toast

Serve small portions every few hours to control diarrhea in young children.

Constipation

Serve lots of liquids! Water, diluted prune juice, noncitrus fruit juices, fruits, and yogurt are good options. For children over one year of age, add a teaspoon of molasses to liquid. Avoid milk products, apples, bananas, rice, or gelatin, as they are binding.

Many well-meaning parents think a child is constipated if there's a bowel movement only every two or three days. But a parent should consider the child's established pattern of bowel movements. A normal frequency ranges from several times a day to once a week. It's better to look at the hardness of the stools rather than their frequency. Small, dry, rocklike stools passed daily or large, firm stools passed once a week (and that clog up the toilet) are both signs of constipation.

Back to Eating

Here are some ideas for coaxing an ailing child back to eating when his or her health returns:

- Offer frequent snacks to disrupt the boredom, encourage small appetites, and increase the intake of fluids and nutrients.
- Allow an "eat where you want" policy.
- Try novelty utensils such as toothpicks.
- Serve foods in tiny portions in muffin tins or egg cartons.
- Place fruit juice in an insulated pitcher at your child's bedside.
- Put soup in a mug.
- Make sandwich faces and cookie-cutter sandwiches.
- Enjoy an indoor picnic on the floor.

Poisons: A Very Real Danger

Always call your poison control center first. If your child is unconscious, call **911**. The phone number for the American Association of Poison Control Centers is **800-222-1222**. Your call will automatically be routed to the poison control center nearest you. Provide as much information as you can, including the child's age, weight, and symptoms, plus when, what, and how much material was ingested.

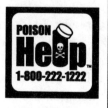

Poisons pose a very real danger to your child. It's a good idea to program the Poison Control number into your home phone and cell phone, or call the 800 number to receive free phone stickers. The hand of a toddler can be quicker than a parent's eye.

Prevention is the best cure. Don't store dangerous materials in low areas, and remember that high places are no longer safe once your child starts climbing. Lock up medicines, household cleaners, paints, lotions, creams, polish, bleach, aspirin, and the like. Don't get in the habit of treating medicine like candy, because it might be eaten that way when you're not around.

Some plants are poisonous, including hyacinth and daffodil bulbs, dieffenbachia (all parts), castor bean (all parts), lily of the valley (leaves and flowers), iris (rhizome), rhubarb leaves (cooked or raw), wild cherries, jack-in-the-pulpit (all parts), and others. Acorns consumed in large quantity can be poisonous; don't let your child chew on them. For a detailed list of plants, see Vicki Lansky's *Baby Proofing Basics* (Book Peddlers) or visit www.vth.colostate.edu/poisonous_plants/report/search.cfm.

The American Academy of Pediatrics (AAP) now encourages parents to discard any syrup of ipecac they currently have at home. Syrup of ipecac is no longer recommended due to its past misuse and uncertain efficacy.

Choking

If your child begins to choke but can breathe (as indicated by coughing or speaking), don't do anything. Encourage your child to cough until the object is cleared. If your child can't breathe (and is younger than one year old), administer five back blows followed by five chest blows. For children older than one year, perform the Heimlich maneuver. To learn how to do these techniques properly, take a local CPR course. It's important to administer them correctly and yet gently enough not to cause internal injuries. Don't practice them at home on your children. Remember, the best treatment for choking is prevention.

And, *finally*, some food for thought from an anonymous author:

How to Bake a Cake

Light oven. Get out bowl, spoons, and ingredients. Grease pan. Crack nuts. Remove 18 blocks and 7 toy autos from kitchen table. Measure 2 cups of flour. Remove Kelly's hands from flour. Wash flour off. Measure 1 more cup of flour to replace flour on floor. Put flour, baking powder, and salt in a sifter. Get dustpan to brush up pieces of bowl Kelly knocked to floor. Get another bowl. Answer phone. Return. Take out greased pan. Remove pinch of salt from pan. Look for Kelly. Get another pan and grease it. Answer phone. Return to kitchen and find Kelly. Remove grimy hands from bowl. Wash off shortening. Take greased pan and find ¼ inch of nutshells in it. Head for Kelly, who flees, knocking bowl off table. Wash kitchen floor, wash table, wash walls, wash dishes, wash Kelly.

Call bakery.
Lie down.

Appendix I:
Weights and Measures

Dairy Substitutes

Baking and run out of milk or cream? Remember that:

If the recipe calls for: *You can substitute:*

1 cup coffee cream   3 tablespoons butter plus ⅞ cup milk

1 cup heavy cream   ⅓ cup butter plus ¾ cup milk

1 cup heavy cream   1 cup reconstituted nonfat dry milk plus
        2½ teaspoons butter or margarine
        or
    ½ cup evaporated milk plus ½ cup water

1 cup buttermilk   1 tablespoon vinegar or lemon juice plus
or juice   enough sweet milk to make 1 cup
        (Let stand 5 minutes before using.)

Substituting Honey for Sugar when Baking

- Use ⅔ cup of honey for each cup of sugar called for.
- For each cup of honey used, subtract about 3 tablespoons of liquid from the recipe. (This does not apply to yeast bread.) In baked goods, add ½ teaspoon soda for every cup substituted.
- Reduce oven temperature by about 25°F and bake a little longer, as honey tends to make baked goods brown faster.
- When using honey instead of brown sugar, use some molasses with the honey.

Size of Can

8 ounces = 1 cup
9 ounces = 1 cup
16 ounces = 2 cups
12 ounces = 1¾ cups
20 ounces (18 fluid) = 2½ cups
28 ounces = 3½ cups
46 ounces = 5¾ cups
6 pounds 10 ounces = 13 cups

Measure for Measure

1 pound flour = 4 cups
1 stick or ¼ pound butter = ½ cup
1 square chocolate = 1 ounce
14 squares graham crackers = 1 cup fine crumbs
1½ slices bread = 1 cup soft crumbs
4 ounces macaroni (1¼ cups) = 2¼ cups cooked
4 ounces noodles (1½–2 cups) = 2 cups cooked
1 cup long-grain rice = 3–4 cups cooked
juice of 1 lemon = 3 tablespoons
grated peel of 1 lemon = 1 teaspoon
juice of 1 orange = ⅓ cup
grated peel of 1 orange = 2 teaspoons
1 medium apple, chopped = 1 cup
1 medium banana, mashed = ⅓ cup
1 pound American cheese, shredded = 4 cups
1 pound raisins = 3½ cups
1 pound carrots = 4 medium or 6 small, 3 cups
  shredded, 2½ cups diced
1 cup milk = ½ cup evaporated milk plus ½ cup water
  OR ⅓ cup dry milk plus 1 cup water
1 cup sour milk = 1 teaspoon vinegar or lemon juice
  plus fresh milk to make 1 cup (Let stand 5 minutes before using.)

Weights and Measures

3 teaspoons = 1 tablespoon
4 tablespoons = ¼ cup
8 tablespoons = ½ cup
16 tablespoons = 1 cup
1 cup = 8 ounces
1 cup = ½ pint
2 cups = 1 pint
2 pints = 1 quart
4 cups = 1 quart
4 quarts = 1 gallon

Appendix II:
Organic Baby Food

Earth's Best (800-434-4246 or www.earthsbest.com)
Healthy Times (877-548-2229 or www.healthytimes.com)
Tender Harvest (800-443-7237 or www.gerber.com)
Nature's Goodness (800-872-2229 or www.naturesgoodness.com)